Speed Learning for Anatomy

SYSTEMS AND FUNCTIONS OF THE HUMAN BODY QUICK AND EASY

Justina C. Bachsteiner PhD

Copyright © 2017 Justina C. Bachsteiner PhD
All rights reserved.

ISBN: 198438581X
ISBN 13: 9781984385819
Library of Congress Control Number: 2018901357
CreateSpace Independent Publishing Platform
North Charleston, South Carolina

Dedicated to my darling daughters
Stephanie, Jessica, and Lauren

Preview

Introduction · ix

Chapters

Chapter 1	The Muscular System ·	1
Chapter 2	The Skeletal System ·	71
Chapter 3	The Digestive System ·	103
Chapter 4	System Integration ·	131
Chapter 5	The Circulatory System ·	231
Chapter 6	The Respiratory System ·	297
Chapter 7	The Nervous System ·	321
Chapter 8	The Integumentary System ·	371
Chapter 9	Tissue Cell Abnormalities ·	405

Table of Contents · xiii

Learn More

Quick Reference to Four Popular Anatomy Categories · 417
Medical Terms · 421
The Four Main Types of Body Tissues · 423
Glossary · 425
Index · 431
Warning · 497

Introduction

<u>Anatomy is a science of classification.</u>

It is a study of the body's structures and the relationships of all the body's parts to one another.

Speed Learning for Anatomy **is a system of learning.**

It is designed to help students reach their learning goals faster and with less effort.

Want to learn faster than ever?

Then this book was written for you.

- You will learn faster because our definitions are brief, accurate, and to the point.

- The writing style is simplistic, nontechnical, and very easy to understand while maintaining a collegiate level of information.

- We utilize a <u>grouping method</u> for terms that are related. For example, when you are looking for the definitions of similar terms, such as *vein* and *artery*, you will see that these terms are grouped together in the same category, which is *blood vessels*. The grouping method enables you to quickly <u>learn each term's definition</u> and <u>compare the differences</u> <u>at a glance</u>. In this category, for example, you will also find the terms: *aorta, coronary arteries, carotid artery, arterioles, capillaries, pulmonary arteries, venous system, vena cava, venules, pulmonary veins, vascular, avascular,* and *lymph*.

- This book contains more than twelve hundred of the most common anatomy terms. Our special grouping method, along with our concise writing style, speeds up your learning by eliminating the usual confusion that is associated with cross-referencing and understanding technical terms.

- What also makes this book so very special is that it is designed for busy students like you who need to learn very quickly. It will be the learning tool that will help you significantly reduce your time studying. The bottom line is when you learn faster, you have more time to learn and more time to devote to other important tasks.

- *Speed Learning for Anatomy* is a compact six-by-nine-inch book that is easy to carry, and it enables you to have the most important anatomy terms readily available at your fingertips.

- Great to keep with you before tests for quick reference, it enables you to review entire anatomy systems in a fraction of the time.

- Great for students, teachers, athletes, fitness trainers, coaches, and all health-conscious people.

- We believe that your learning experience needs to be <u>as painless as possible</u>, and that is why our dedicated goal is to present you with the most helpful learning tool available: <u>this book</u>!

We go the extra mile!

- Images have been added to help you understand written concepts and explanations.

- We are <u>intentionally</u> stepping outside the usual scope of anatomy books by including <u>practical</u> information about *your body* that you can apply to *your life*.

If you study it, why not learn how to apply it?

We've expanded this scope to include:

- Aerobic calculations
- Aerobic training guidelines
- Stretch response
- Health conditions
    - Cancer
    - Diabetes
    - Heart Conditions
- Body-building charts and guidelines
- Eye Anatomy
- Vitamin and mineral descriptions
- Medical terms, and much more

In *Speed Learning for Anatomy* you will not only learn basic anatomy, <u>but also how to apply your acquired knowledge to enhance your own life</u>.

- You won't find this kind of accurate, scientific information in other anatomy books. For example:

    - You will learn about the many functions of muscle tissue and then learn how best to develop your own muscle composition. We've even included workout charts explaining what machines to use for each muscle group.

    - We've included simplified formulas for heart rate and aerobic calculations, such as
        - Karvonen Formula
        - VO2 Max
        - Maximum/Maximal Aerobic Capacity
        - Maximum/Maximal Oxygen Consumption
        - Maximum Heart Rate (MHR)

    - We've chosen to discuss some of <u>the most common health conditions</u> simply because they are part of the human condition <u>and are always related to our anatomy</u>. Awareness and understanding of health conditions have unlimited benefits.

- This book is all about giving you every benefit we can offer to your scholastic endeavors, as well as the life you live.

Speed Learning for Anatomy gives you a tremendous learning advantage. The following nine chapters define a vast array of information relating to anatomy. The definitions are crisp, to the point, and designed for you to understand concepts quickly and easily. Simplifying anatomy terms and saving you valuable learning time is what makes this book so special.

No other anatomy book defines anatomy terms so clearly, or so simply.

Table of Contents

Introduction · ix

Chapter 1 The Muscular System · 1
   1.1 Anatomy of the Muscular System · 3
      1.1.1 Introduction to the Muscular System · · · · · · · · · · · · · · · · · · · 5
      1.1.2 Types of Muscle Tissue · 6
      1.1.3 Skeletal Muscles · 8
      1.1.4 Types of Skeletal Muscle Fiber · 10
      1.1.5 Muscle Fiber Composition and Function · · · · · · · · · · · · · · · · 12
      1.1.6 Additional Structures of Skeletal Muscle · · · · · · · · · · · · · · · · 14
      1.1.7 Muscle Characteristics · 16
      1.1.8 Neuromuscular System · 23
      1.1.9 Synovial Joint Motions and the Muscles Involved · · · · · · · · · · · 25
      1.1.10 Major Skeletal Muscles and Their Joint Motions · · · · · · · · · · · · 29
      1.1.11 Connective Tissue Types · 36

   1.2 Stretching & Flexibility · 39
      1.2.1 Muscle Stretching vs. Muscle Contraction and Stabilization · · 41
      1.2.2 Flexibility of Joints · 42
      1.2.3 Flexibility of Connective Tissue · 43
      1.2.4 Types of Stretching · 44
      1.2.5 Neurophysiological Effects of Stretching · · · · · · · · · · · · · · · · · · 48
      1.2.6 Safety Responses to Muscle Contraction & Muscle
             Stretching · 50

   1.3 Musculoskeletal Injuries and Conditions · 53
      1.3.1 Common Musculoskeletal Injuries and Conditions · · · · · · · · · 55
      1.3.2 Common Leg Injuries and Conditions · 60
      1.3.3 Overstretching (Stretch Weakness) · 65
      1.3.4 Techniques Used to Treat Muscle Injury (RICE) · · · · · · · · · · · · · 66
      1.3.5 Muscular System Testing Devices · 68

Chapter 2 The Skeletal System ·71
   2.1 Anatomy of the Skeletal System ·73
      2.1.1 Skeletal Categories and Functions ·75
      2.1.2 Standard Anatomical Position ·76
      2.1.3 Axial Skeleton ·78
      2.1.4 Appendicular Skeleton ·79
      2.1.5 Bones of the Skull ·80
      2.1.6 Bones of the Vertebral Column ·82
      2.1.7 Joints ·84
      2.1.8 Three Primary Joints Types ·85
      2.1.9 Anatomical Planes ·86
      2.1.10 Synovial Joint Motions ·88
      2.1.11 Mechanics of Synovial Joints ·91

   2.2 Skeletal System Injuries and Conditions ·93
      2.2.1 Arthritis ·95
      2.2.2 Stress Fracture ·99
      2.2.3 Posture Abnormalities ·100
      2.2.4 Cortisone for Pain Relief ·101

Chapter 3 The Digestive System ·· 103
   3.1   Anatomy of the Digestive System ······························ 105
       3.1.1   Gastrointestinal Tract ··· 107
       3.1.2   Small Intestine ·· 110
       3.1.3   Large Intestine ·· 112
       3.1.4   Additional Digestive System Components ················ 113

   3.2   Digestive System Injuries and Conditions ···················· 117
       3.2.1   Hernia ·· 119
       3.2.2   Peptic Ulcer ·· 121
       3.2.3   Irritable Bowel Syndrome (IBS) ···························· 122
       3.2.4   Hemorrhoids ·· 124
       3.2.5   Crohn's Disease ··· 126
       3.2.6   Acid Reflux ··· 129

Chapter 4 System Integration ··· 131
    4.1 Body Composition and Energy Systems ······················· 133
        4.1.1   What Body Weight Reveals and What It Doesn't ··········· 135
        4.1.2   Body Fat ··· 137
        4.1.3   Types of Fat Cells ·· 138
        4.1.4   What is the "Best" Way to Lose Body Fat? ················· 139
        4.1.5   How Many Calories Do I Need to Cut to Lose Weight? ····· 141
        4.1.6   Eating Disorders ··· 143
        4.1.7   Calorie Burning Comparison for Exercise ················· 147
        4.1.8   Effect of Muscle Size on Lean Body Mass ················· 149
        4.1.9   Calories Burned by Adding Muscle ························ 150
        4.1.10 Body Weight Stabilization ·································· 152
        4.1.11 Body Function Stabilization ································ 154
        4.1.12 Health Conditions Resulting from Chemical Imbalances ··· 156
        4.1.13 Metabolism ··· 158
        4.1.14 Basal Metabolic Rate (BMR) ································ 159
        4.1.15 Energy Sources ··· 161
        4.1.16 Diabetes Mellitus and Hypoglycemia ····················· 165
        4.1.17 Aerobic and Anaerobic-Energy Systems ·················· 167
        4.1.18 Body Mass Index (BMI) ······································ 169
        4.1.19 BMI Formula ·· 170
        4.1.20 BMI Range Chart for Weight Categories ·················· 172
        4.1.21 Understanding Body Fat Percentage ······················ 173

    4.2 Body Building ·· 175
        4.2.1   How to Build Muscle Size and Strength ··················· 177
        4.2.2   Basic Muscle-Building Workout Charts ···················· 179
        4.2.3   Benefits of Warm-Ups and Cool-Downs ··················· 181
        4.2.4   Are "Spot Reducing" Exercises Effective? ·················· 183
        4.2.5   Exercise Increases Abdominal Definition ················· 184
        4.2.6   Heat Conditions ·· 185
        4.2.7   Wolff's Law ·· 188

4.3 Nutrition · 189

- 4.3.1 Calories and Kilocalories · 191
- 4.3.2 Caloric Values of the Three Main Nutrient Groups · · · · · · · · · 192
- 4.3.3 Essential Nutrients · 193
- 4.3.4 Nutrient Density · 194
- 4.3.5 Six Nutrient Categories · 195
- 4.3.6 Symbols that Express the Quantities of Nutrients · · · · · · · · · · · 196
- 4.3.7 Suggested Daily Intakes · 197
- 4.3.8 Water · 198
- 4.3.9 Carbohydrates · 199
- 4.3.10 Muscles & Protein · 203
- 4.3.11 Amino Acids · 205
- 4.3.12 Essential and Nonessential Amino Acids · 206
- 4.3.13 Fat and Fatty Acids · 207
- 4.3.14 Three Main Types of Fatty Acids · 209
- 4.3.15 Essential Fatty Acids · 211
- 4.3.16 "Bad" Fats · 213
- 4.3.17 Dietary Fat Intake · 215
- 4.3.18 Vitamins and Minerals · 217
- 4.3.19 Vitamin Descriptions · 220
- 4.3.20 Mineral Descriptions · 225
- 4.3.21 Free Radicals, Antioxidants, and CoQ10 · 228
- 4.3.22 Phytochemicals (Plant Chemicals) · 230

Chapter 5 The Circulatory System ··· 231
    5.1 Anatomy of the Circulatory System ·························· 233
        5.1.1 Components of the Circulatory System ·················· 235
        5.1.2 Heart ·· 237
        5.1.3 Structure of the Heart ···································· 239
        5.1.4 Layers of the Heart Wall ·································· 240
        5.1.5 Heart Chambers ··· 241
        5.1.6 The Heart Map ·· 243
        5.1.7 Diagnosing Circulatory Sounds ·························· 245
        5.1.8 Blood Pressure ·· 247
        5.1.9 Pulse ·· 248
        5.1.10 Cardio Measurements ··································· 249
        5.1.11 Blood Function ··· 251
        5.1.12 Blood Components ····································· 252
        5.1.13 Types of Blood Vessels ·································· 254
        5.1.14 Circulatory System - Image ······························ 258

    5.2 Heart Healthy Exercise ··· 259
        5.2.1 Ergometer ··· 261
        5.2.2 Cardio Endurance ······································ 262
        5.2.3 The Capacity to Consume Oxygen ······················ 263
        5.2.4 Aerobic Training Guidelines (Beginners) ················· 264
        5.2.5 MET System ··· 271
        5.2.6 Maximum Heart Rate and Calculations ·················· 273
        5.2.7 Maximum Heart Rate Compared to Aerobic Capacity ····· 275
        5.2.8 Karvonen Formula ······································ 276
        5.2.9 Karvonen Formula Calculations ························· 277
        5.2.10 Using the Karvonen Formula ···························· 278
        5.2.11 How to Train Safely ····································· 280

5.3 Circulatory System Injuries and Conditions ·283
    5.3.1 Heart Conditions ·285
    5.3.2 Blood Conditions ·288
    5.3.3 Understanding Cholesterol ·289
    5.3.4 Cholesterol Terms ·290
    5.3.5 Cholesterol Range References ·292
    5.3.6 Dietary Fat and Cholesterol Levels ·293
    5.3.7 Blood Vessel Conditions ·295

Chapter 6 The Respiratory System ·· 297
    6.1 Anatomy of the Respiratory System ···························· 299
        6.1.1 Respiratory System ··· 301
        6.1.2 Airway Components·· 304
        6.1.3 Pulmonary Blood Vessels ··································· 310
        6.1.4 Muscles Used for Breathing ······························· 311

    6.2 Respiratory System Injuries and Conditions ················ 315
        6.2.1 Respiratory Conditions ···································· 317
        6.2.2 Breathing Abnormalities ·································· 319

Chapter 7 The Nervous System · 321
7.1 Anatomy of the Nervous System · 323
7.1.1   Nervous System Divisions · 325
7.1.2   Subdivisions of the Central Nervous System · · · · · · · · · · · · · · · 327
7.1.3   Subdivisions of the Peripheral Nervous System · · · · · · · · · · · · 328
7.1.4   Brain Anatomy · 330
7.1.5   Left and Right Brain Functions · 332
7.1.6   Structure of a Typical Neuron · 333
7.1.7   Brain Wave and Electrical Activity Testing · · · · · · · · · · · · · · · · · 336
7.1.8   Anatomy of the Spinal Cord · 337
7.1.9   Eyes and Nervous System · 342
7.1.10 Components of Eye Anatomy · 343
7.1.11 Eye Function · 349

7.2 Nervous System Injuries and Conditions · 351
7.2.1   Seizures (Convulsions) · 353
7.2.2   Health Conditions of the Nervous System · · · · · · · · · · · · · · · · · 355
7.2.3   Arthritis Types That May Affect the Spine · · · · · · · · · · · · · · · · · 358
7.2.4   Acquired Causes of Spinal Conditions · 359
7.2.5   Eye Conditions · 362
7.2.6   Eye Tests · 365
7.2.7   Eye Surgery and Treatments · 367

Chapter 8 The Integumentary System ··371
    8.1   Anatomy of the Integumentary System························373
        8.1.1   Skin ··375
        8.1.2   Skin Layers ···376
        8.1.3   Skin Cells··378
        8.1.4   Exocrine Glands and Endocrine Glands····················379
        8.1.5   Sweat Glands··382
        8.1.6   Mammary Glands ···383
        8.1.7   Ear Glands···384
        8.1.8   Types of Hair ···385
        8.1.9   Hair Functions··386
        8.1.10 Nails ···387

    8.2   Integumentary System Injuries and Conditions ···············389
        8.2.1   Skin Conditions···391
        8.2.2   Common Adverse Skin Reactions ·························394
        8.2.3   Burns··395
        8.2.4   Types of Skin Wounds ······································396
        8.2.5   Bleeding··397
        8.2.6   Symptoms···398
        8.2.7   Types of Blisters···400
        8.2.8   Scar Tissue ··401
        8.2.9   Ear Condition ···402
        8.2.10 Hair and Scalp Conditions ································403
        8.2.11 Cosmetic Surgery···404

Chapter 9 Tissue Cell Abnormalities ···405
    9.1   Tissue Cell Abnormalities ·······································407
        9.1.1   Cancer Conditions ··409
        9.1.2   Body Types and Growth Abnormalities ····················414

CHAPTER 1

The Muscular System

1.1 Anatomy of the Muscular System ································ 3
    1.1.1 Introduction to the Muscular System ···················· 5
    1.1.2 Types of Muscle Tissue ································ 6
    1.1.3 Skeletal Muscles ···································· 8
    1.1.4 Types of Skeletal Muscle Fiber ························ 10
    1.1.5 Muscle Fiber Composition and Function ················ 12
    1.1.6 Additional Structures of Skeletal Muscle ················ 14
    1.1.7 Muscle Characteristics ······························ 16
    1.1.8 Neuromuscular System ······························ 23
    1.1.9 Synovial Joint Motions and the Muscles Involved ········· 25
    1.1.10 Major Skeletal Muscles and Their Joint Motions ········· 29
    1.1.11 Connective Tissue Types ···························· 36

1.2 Stretching & Flexibility ···································· 39
    1.2.1 Muscle Stretching vs. Muscle Contraction and Stabilization ·· 41
    1.2.2 Flexibility of Joints ································· 42
    1.2.3 Flexibility of Connective Tissue ······················· 43
    1.2.4 Types of Stretching ································· 44
    1.2.5 Neurophysiological Effects of Stretching ················ 48
    1.2.6 Safety Responses to Muscle Contraction & Muscle Stretching ··· 50

1.3 Musculoskeletal Injuries and Conditions ······················ 53
    1.3.1 Common Musculoskeletal Injuries and Conditions ········ 55
    1.3.2 Common Leg Injuries and Conditions ·················· 60
    1.3.3 Overstretching (Stretch Weakness) ···················· 65
    1.3.4 Techniques Used to Treat Muscle Injury (RICE) ··········· 66
    1.3.5 Muscular System Testing Devices ····················· 68

1.1 Anatomy of the Muscular System

1.1.1

Introduction to the Muscular System

- **Number of Muscles**
- **Muscle Function**
- **Muscle Components**

There are more than six hundred muscles within the human body and more than 430 are voluntary muscles. Muscles are responsible for a great variety of functions, including body motion, strength, posture, heat production, and much more. Muscle is composed of approximately 75 percent water, 20 percent protein, and 5 percent salts and other chemicals.

1.1.2

Types of Muscle Tissue

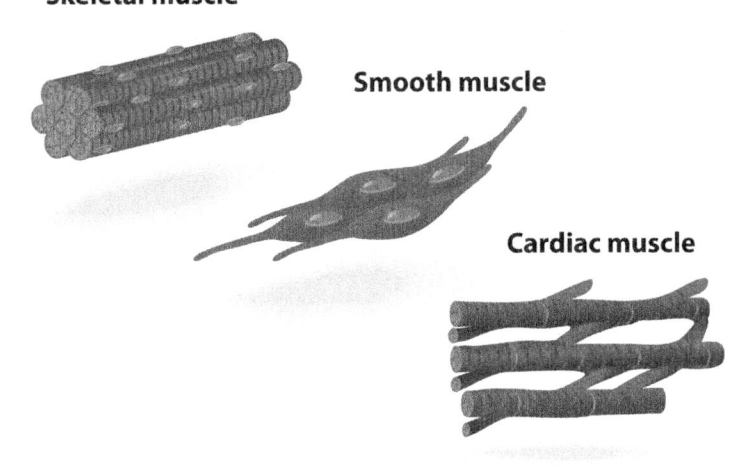

1. Skeletal Muscle (Voluntary Muscle Tissues)
2. Smooth Muscle (Involuntary Muscle Tissues)
3. Cardiac Muscle (Involuntary Muscle Tissues)

Skeletal Muscle
- Skeletal muscles form the muscles of the arms, legs, chest, back, neck, and head. They are primarily responsible for body movements.
- These tissues are <u>voluntary</u> because they are under conscious control.
- The skeletal muscles also have other important functions, including the ability to increase basal metabolic rates (BMR), store energy, add body strength, and improve body appearance.
- By increasing muscle size and strength, bones simultaneously get stronger and denser.
- All the skeletal muscles are attached to the bones by connective tissues called tendons.

Smooth Muscle
- Smooth muscle, also called <u>visceral muscles</u>, help to form the walls of certain internal organs, such as the esophagus, the stomach, the intestines, and blood vessels.
- These tissues are <u>involuntary</u> because they are not considered to be under conscious control.

Cardiac Muscle
- Cardiac muscle is comprised of involuntary muscle tissues that form the walls of the heart muscle.
- These tissues are <u>involuntary</u> because they are not considered to be under conscious control.

1.1.3

Skeletal Muscles

Front & Side View

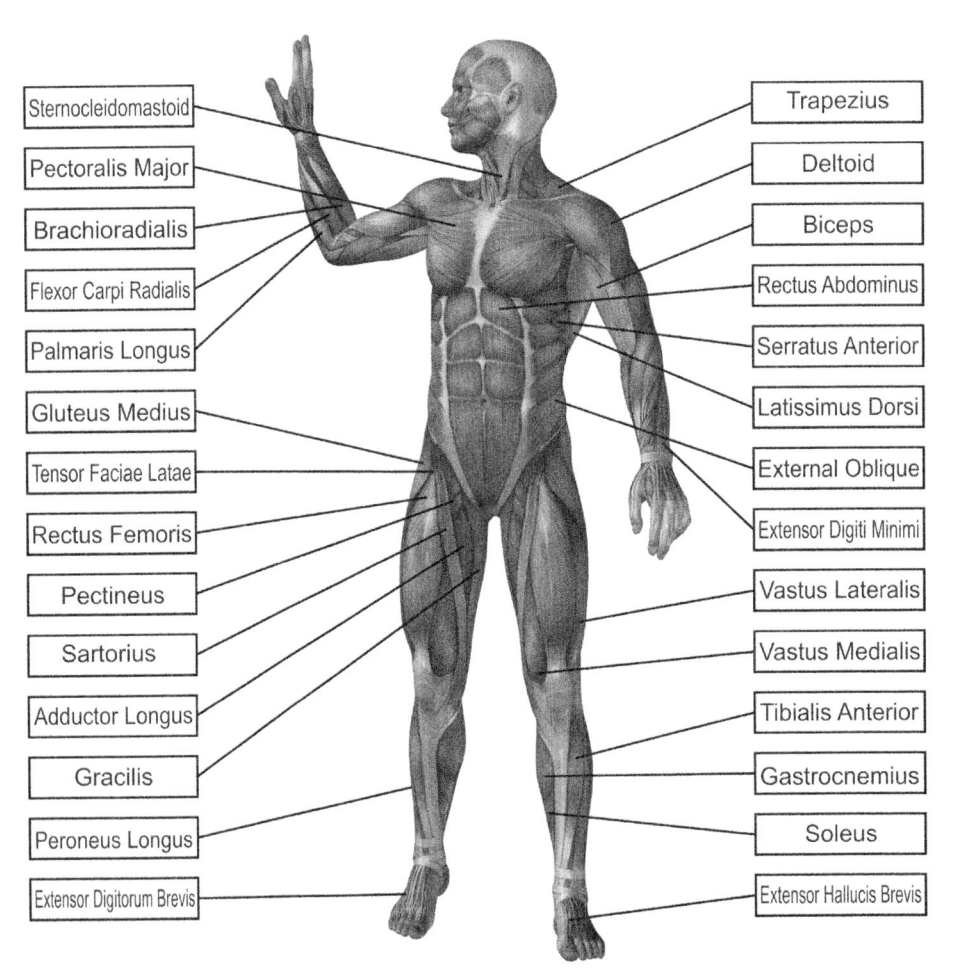

- Sternocleidomastoid
- Pectoralis Major
- Brachioradialis
- Flexor Carpi Radialis
- Palmaris Longus
- Gluteus Medius
- Tensor Faciae Latae
- Rectus Femoris
- Pectineus
- Sartorius
- Adductor Longus
- Gracilis
- Peroneus Longus
- Extensor Digitorum Brevis

- Trapezius
- Deltoid
- Biceps
- Rectus Abdominus
- Serratus Anterior
- Latissimus Dorsi
- External Oblique
- Extensor Digiti Minimi
- Vastus Lateralis
- Vastus Medialis
- Tibialis Anterior
- Gastrocnemius
- Soleus
- Extensor Hallucis Brevis

SPEED LEARNING FOR ANATOMY

Back View

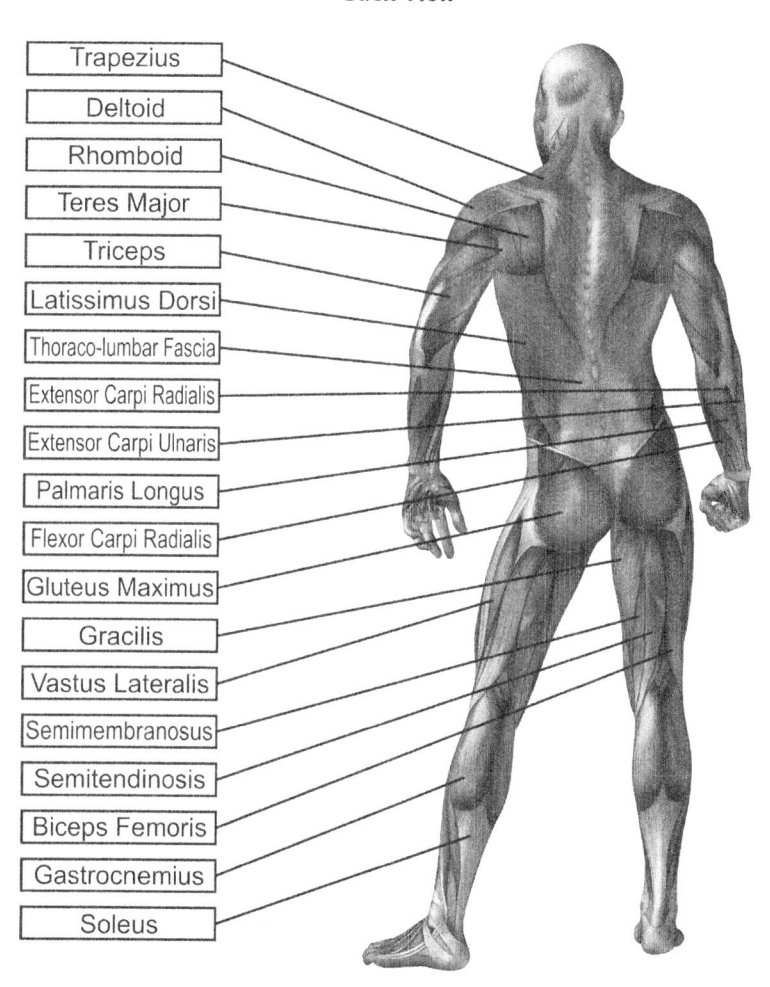

- Trapezius
- Deltoid
- Rhomboid
- Teres Major
- Triceps
- Latissimus Dorsi
- Thoraco-lumbar Fascia
- Extensor Carpi Radialis
- Extensor Carpi Ulnaris
- Palmaris Longus
- Flexor Carpi Radialis
- Gluteus Maximus
- Gracilis
- Vastus Lateralis
- Semimembranosus
- Semitendinosis
- Biceps Femoris
- Gastrocnemius
- Soleus

1.1.4

Types of Skeletal Muscle Fiber

- Fast-twitch White Muscle Fiber
- Slow-twitch Red Muscle Fiber
- Distribution of Muscle Fiber

Fast- and slow-twitch muscle fibers (cells) are only present in the skeletal muscles.

Fast-twitch White Muscle Fiber
- Also called Type 2 muscle fiber, this type of fiber is good for anaerobic activity, such as weight lifting, and is characterized by its fast speed of contraction and its high capacity for anaerobic glycolysis.
- People with greater percentages of fast-twitch fiber have more strength for anaerobic activity. These people also develop muscle strength and size faster than those with less fast-twitch fiber.
- Professional-level power athletes, such as power weight lifters, have a fast-twitch fiber distribution of approximately 60–90 percent in the muscles used for their sport.

Slow-twitch <u>Red</u> Muscle Fiber
- Also called <u>Type 1 muscle fiber</u>, this type of fiber is good for <u>aerobic activity,</u> such as running, and is characterized by its <u>slow speed of contraction</u> and a <u>high capacity for aerobic glycolysis.</u>
- People with greater percentages of slow-twitch fiber have more endurance for aerobic activity.
- Professional-level endurance athletes, such as cross-country skiers and runners, have a slow-twitch fiber distribution of approximately 60–90 percent in the muscles used for their sport.

Distribution of Muscle Fiber
- Muscle fiber distribution is entirely genetic.
- Training will not change one fiber type to another fiber type.
- <u>Male muscle tissue is not any stronger than female muscle tissue</u>. It's just that men usually have <u>more</u> muscle tissue.
- A male fast-twitch fiber is no different from a female fast-twitch fiber. Also, male slow-twitch fiber is no different from female slow-twitch fiber.

1.1.5

Muscle Fiber Composition and Function

- Nucleus
- Sarcolemma
- Mitochondria
- Myofibril
- Sliding Filament Theory

Muscle Fiber

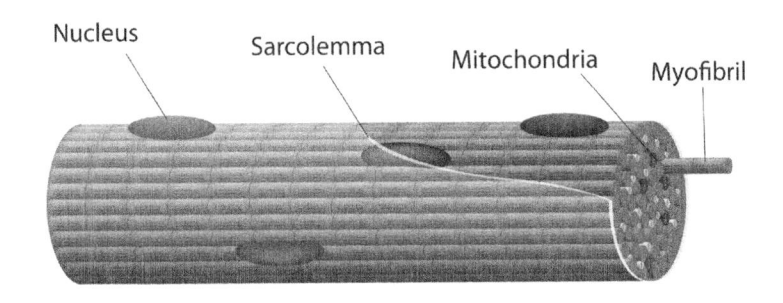

Nucleus — Sarcolemma — Mitochondria — Myofibril

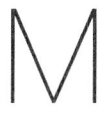

Muscles are composed of large numbers of muscle fibers (sometimes referred to as muscle cells) that have the following components:

Nucleus
- The structure in a cell that contains the chromosomes.
- The nucleus has a membrane around it and is where RNA is made from the DNA in the chromosomes.

Sarcolemma
- The plasma membrane of skeletal muscle (and cardiac muscle) cells.

Mitochondria

The sites of <u>aerobic</u> ATP energy production. ATP, or *adenosine triphosphate* is a high-energy phosphate molecule that is necessary to supply energy for cell function. It is stored in the muscles and produced both <u>aerobically and anaerobically</u>. The sites of <u>anaerobic</u> ATP energy production are inside the cells but <u>outside the mitochondria</u>.

Myofibril
- <u>Strands of contractile proteins</u> situated throughout the length of a muscle fiber.
- Though other proteins are present in a myofibril, there are only <u>two types of contractile proteins</u>:
    1. Actin
    2. Myosin
- These proteins run through all the <u>sarcomeres</u> (repeating units of muscle fibers along the length of the muscle cell) that are necessary for <u>muscle contraction</u>.
    - Myofibrils increase in <u>number and size</u> with strength training.
    - Sarcomeres increase in <u>number</u> with strength training.

Sliding Filament Theory
- This theory states that there must be an <u>interaction</u> between the <u>energy from ATP</u> and the <u>contractile proteins</u> (actin and myosin) and must include a <u>nervous impulse from the Central Nervous System</u> to cause muscles to contract.

1.1.6

Additional Structures of Skeletal Muscle

- **Endomysium**
- **Fascicles**
- **Perimysium**
- **EpimysiumTendons**

Structure of Skeletal Muscle

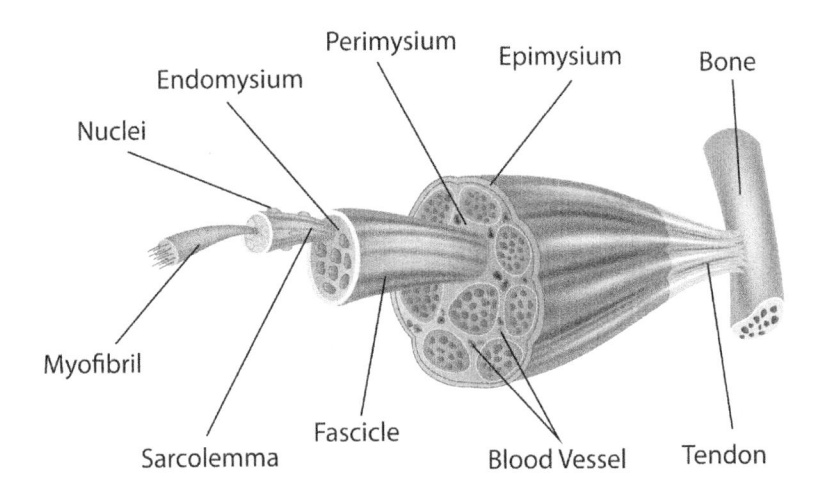

Interdependent Contracting Skeletal Muscle Fibers
- In order for contracting skeletal muscle fibers to be functional, they **cannot** work as independent or isolated units. It is necessary for them to be bound together.
- Every skeletal muscle fiber is bound to its adjacent fiber by the **endomysium** to form bundles called **fascicles**.
- Neighboring fascicles are bound together by another type of connective sheath called the **perimysium**.
- The final outer sheath of the entire muscle group is the **epimysium,** which is continuous with **tendons** that attach the muscle to bone.

1.1.7

Muscle Characteristics

- <u>Muscle Size:</u>
    - Hypertrophy
        - Sarcomere
    - Hyperplasia
    - Atrophy
- <u>Muscle Contraction:</u>
    - Muscle Force
    - Isometric
    - Concentric
    - Eccentric
- <u>Muscle Attachment</u>
    - Proximal
    - Distal
    - Origin
    - Tendon Insertion
- <u>Muscle Stabilization:</u>
    - Agonist
    - Antagonist
    - Synergist

Muscle Size

Hypertrophy
- <u>An increase in muscle fiber size</u> resulting in strength gains and muscle size.
- <u>A person cannot increase their number of muscle fibers</u>, only the size and strength of their muscle fibers.
- Muscles get bigger and stronger only by <u>necessity</u>.
- <u>Strength training</u> is the only way to significantly increase muscle size and strength.
    - Regular strength training signals to the muscles that they need to accommodate the burden of lifting heavier weight, and they respond by growing in size and strength.
    - Technically, <u>hypertrophy results from an increase in the number and size of myofibrils</u> inside a muscle fiber, resulting in increases to muscle strength and size.
    - Another way to describe hypertrophy is an increase in the <u>amount of the contractile proteins</u> (actin and myosin).

Sarcomere
- An additional benefit of <u>strength training</u> is an increase in *sarcomeres* (See 1.1.5 <u>Muscle Fiber Composition and Function</u> and then look under <u>Myofibril</u>).

- While most men desire an increase in muscle size and strength, it is not quite as favored by many women due to their concern about developing a "body builder's" body. The fact is that most women cannot develop a high level of muscle size due to their naturally low levels of testosterone.

- <u>Best ages for the rate of strength gain</u> are between the ages of ten to twenty, the years of normal growth and development.

- However, men and women of all ages can increase muscle size and strength with progressive strength training.

Hyperplasia
- An increase in the number of muscle fibers.
- There is no credible evidence that hyperplasia is possible in humans.

Atrophy
- A decrease in muscle size and strength.
- Causes are inactivity or immobilization resulting from an injury, age, or illness.

Muscle Contraction

- Muscles never push; they always pull.
- In any given action between two bones, one bone is generally in a fixed position, and the other bone has motion.
- The action is always the result of muscle contraction or, to say it another way, the involved muscle pulling.

Muscle Force
- When a skeletal muscle fiber contracts, it creates force.
- It functions on an **all or none principle:**
  - This means that it exerts its maximum force automatically.
  - It cannot regulate the force it produces, as can cardiac muscle fiber.
- The force a **single muscle fiber** creates during contraction is directly related to its size.
- Larger fiber means greater force.
- The amount of force an **entire muscle creates** during contraction is directly related to:
  - The size of the fibers within the muscle.
  - The number of fibers within the muscle that contract simultaneously.

Isometric Contraction
- In this type of contraction, the applied muscular force is <u>equal to</u> the resistive force (*an external force that resists the motion of another force*) and the result is no movement.
- A typical example of isometric contraction is when a person places his hands in front of his chest and presses the palms together with equal force, resulting in no body movement. <u>Muscle fibers contract, but muscle length remains constant.</u>

Concentric Contraction
- In this type of contraction, the applied muscular force is <u>greater than</u> the resistive force and the <u>muscle shortens</u> as its fibers <u>contract</u> to overcome the resistance.
- A typical example would be the <u>lifting phase</u> (positive phase) of a biceps curl.

Eccentric Contraction
- In this type of contraction, the applied muscular force is <u>less than</u> the resistive force and the <u>muscle lengthens</u> as its fibers <u>contract</u> to overcome the resistance.
- A typical example would be the <u>lowering phase</u> (negative phase) of a biceps curl.

Reviewing Muscle Contraction (<u>Concentric vs. Eccentric</u>)

Contraction Types:	**Opposite Reactions:**	**Same Reactions:**
1. *Concentric* Contraction	Muscle *shortens*	Fibers *contract*
2. *Eccentric* Contraction	Muscle *lengthens*	Fibers *contract*

- **Muscles always pull; they never push,** regardless of how the body motion appears.

- For example, when a person is **pushing furniture** along the floor or performing **push-ups,** the muscles involved contract concentrically, causing the muscles to shorten, while the muscle fibers simultaneously contract.

- In both examples, the concentric contraction of the triceps, chest, and shoulder muscles, acting together, force the arms to move forward to push.

Muscle Attachment

Muscle Attachment Relating to a Limb
- **Proximal**
  - The direction that is toward the attached end of a limb, closest to the head.

- **Distal (a)**
  - The direction that is away from the attached end of a limb, furthest from the head.

Muscle Attachment Relating to a Motion
- **Origin**
  - The site of muscle attachment to the fixed bone.

- **Distal (b)**
  - The site of muscle attachment to the bone that has motion.

Tendon Insertion
- The location of the tendon insertion has an effect on muscle strength.
- As an example:
  - Mary and Joan have identical biceps strength, biceps length, and forearm length.
  - However, Mary's biceps tendon attaches (the insertion point) further down her forearm, and therefore further from her elbow than Joan's biceps tendon.
  - The location of Mary's tendon insertion gives her a biomechanical advantage.
  - It enables her to apply more strength to elbow flexion exercises such as a biceps curl.

Muscle Stabilization

- In general, muscles stabilize one joint in order to enable another joint to perform a desired motion.
- A typical example of the action of stabilizer muscles is when both the *latissimus dorsi* (back muscles) and the *pectoralis major* (chest muscles) contract isometrically, and simultaneously, for the purpose of stabilizing the shoulder joint in order to enable the elbow joint to be flexed when performing a proper form biceps curl.
- It should be noted that many isolated exercises (exercises that are properly performed only when there is no motion at other joints, such as the biceps curl, leg curl, and leg extension) require the stabilization of other joints.

Agonist Muscle
- Most muscles of the trunk and the extremities exist in opposing pairs. When one muscle of the pair contracts to create a desired motion, that muscle is called the agonist muscle. As this contraction occurs, an opposite muscle of the same pair, called the antagonist muscle (see below), stretches.
- For example, when the biceps muscle is contracted, the tricep muscle simultaneously stretches. In this example, the contracting biceps muscle is the agonist, and the stretching triceps muscle is the antagonist.

Antagonist Muscle
- The antagonist muscle is always the muscle that opposes the action of the agonist muscle. Additionally, <u>the antagonist muscle is always the muscle that is stretching</u>, while, conversely, the agonist muscle is always contracting.

Synergist Muscles
- The combined function of <u>two or more muscles acting together</u> to perform an anatomical movement is referred to as synergistic.
- For example, when performing a leg extension exercise, there are four muscles that act together (as synergists) to enable the leg to do this exercise. These four muscles, known collectively as the **quadriceps,** are the:
    1. *Rectus femoris*
    2. *Vastus lateralis*
    3. *Vastus medialis*
    4. *Vastus intermedius*

1.1.8

Neuromuscular System

- **Motor Unit**
- **Motor Neuron**
- **Motor Learning Factor**
- **Nervous Inhibition**

Neuromuscular System
- The network of nerves that is responsible for the contraction or relaxation of muscles, including the muscle fibers that are connected to them.

Motor Unit
- Located within a muscle, it is a single motor nerve, and all the muscle fibers that it stimulates.
- Motor units can also exist in groups.
- Motor units vary in size:
  - A small motor unit can have a nerve that activates only five to ten muscle fibers.
  - These units are responsible for such delicate actions as blinking, or using a tweezer.
  - A large motor unit can have a nerve that activates 500–1000 muscle fibers.
  - These units are responsible for such actions as lifting, going up steps, or any activity that requires effort.
- Motor units are made of either:
  - All fast twitch muscle fibers, or,
  - All slow twitch muscle fibers.
  - When fibers of a muscle unit contract, every fiber in that unit contracts simultaneously, and with maximum force (the all or none principle).
  - Force generated is relative to the amount of motor units that are stimulated to contract simultaneously.
  (See Muscle Force in Section 1.1.7 Muscle Characteristics)

Motor Neuron
- A <u>nerve cell</u> that carries motor commands from the central nervous system to the muscles and glands of the body.
- These commands act as messages that direct the muscles and glands to function in a way that is most beneficial to the body.

Motor Learning Factor
- A significant amount of the strength gains that occur in the very early phases of strength training are due to <u>improved neurological factors (motor learning)</u>, as opposed to the development of larger muscle fibers.
- However, as strength training continues, strength gains are related more and more to the development of larger muscle fibers.

Nervous Inhibition
- Comprised of both physiological and psychological components, nervous inhibition negatively affects the muscles by inhibiting developmental progress.
- **From a psychological standpoint,** nervous inhibition is a lack of confidence that restricts the individual's willingness to apply optimal physical performance.
- **From a physiological standpoint**, nervous inhibition reduces physical effort resulting in lessened muscle development.

1.1.9

Synovial Joint Motions and the Muscles Involved

- Charts 1–3 below list the <u>muscles involved in synovial joint motions, or diarthrosis</u>.

- <u>Most of the joints of the body</u> are synovial joints, which make up the largest functional category of joints in the body.

- <u>Synovial joints have a joint cavity</u> and fibrous connective tissue. Examples include the shoulder, elbow, hip, knee and ankle.

- Many different types of motions occur at various synovial joint locations throughout the body.

See the following pages for:
- Types of Synovial Joint Motions
- Muscles Involved
    - Chart 1: Shoulder and Elbow
    - Chart 2: Hip
    - Chart 3: Knee and Ankle

Chart 1: Shoulder and Elbow

Types of Synovial Joint Motions	Muscles Involved
Shoulder flexion	Biceps brachii Anterior deltoid Coracobrachialis Pectoralis major
Shoulder extension	Posterior deltoid Triceps Latissimus dorsi Teres major
Shoulder abduction	Middle deltoid Supraspinatus
Shoulder adduction	Pectoralis major Latissimus dorsi Teres major
Shoulder medial rotation	Latissimus dorsi Teres major
Shoulder lateral rotation	Infraspinatus Teres minor
Shoulder transverse adduction	Pectoralis major Coracobrachialis Anterior deltoid
Shoulder transverse abduction	Triceps Posterior deltoid
Elbow flexion	Biceps brachii Brachialis Brachioradialis
Elbow extension	Triceps

Chart 2: Hip

Types of Synovial Joint Motions	Muscles Involved
Hip flexion	*Iliopsoas* *Rectus femoris* *Sartorius*
Hip extension	*Gluteus maximus* *Biceps femoris* *Semitendinosus* *Semimembranosus*
Hip abduction	*Tensor fasciae latae* *Gluteus medius* *Gluteus minimus*
Hip adduction	*Pectineus* *Adductor longus* *Adductor magnus* *Adductor brevis* *Gracilis*
Hip lateral rotation	*Six internal rotators* *Gluteus maximus*
Hip medial rotation	*Iliopsoas* *Tensor fasciae latae*

Chart 3: Knee and Ankle

Types of Synovial Joint Motions	Muscles Involved
Knee flexion	*Biceps femoris* *Semitendinosus* *Semimembranosus* *Sartorius*
Knee extension	*Rectus femoris* *Vastus lateralis* *Vastus medialis* *Vastus intermedius*
Ankle dorsiflexion	*Tibialis anterior* *Extensor digitorum longus*
Ankle plantar flexion	*Gastrocnemius* *Soleus* *Tibialis posterior* *Flexor digitorum longus* *Flexor hallucis longus* *Peroneus longus and brevis* *Peroneus tertius*

1.1.10

Major Skeletal Muscles and Their Joint Motions

- The following muscles, or groups of muscles, contract concentrically to create movement at a joint. That is, the applied muscular force is <u>greater than</u> the resistive force.
- <u>Muscle length shortens</u> as its fibers <u>contract</u> to overcome the resistance.

For example:
- The biceps contract concentrically to flex the upper arm.
- The quadriceps contract concentrically to extend the leg.

See the following pages for:
- Major Skeletal Muscles of the Body
- Groups of Muscles That Form Each Skeletal Muscle
- Primary Joint Motions
    - Chart 1: Legs
    - Chart 2: Buttocks & Abdominals
    - Chart 3: Back
    - Chart 4: Chest & Shoulders
    - Chart 5: Biceps & Triceps
    - Chart 6: Forearms & Wrist

Chart 1: Legs

Major Skeletal Muscles of the Body	Groups of Muscles That Form Each Skeletal Muscle	Primary Joint Motions
Legs (Quadriceps)	1. *Rectus femoris* 2. *Vastus medialis* 3. *Vastus intermedius* 4. *Vastus lateralis*	Extension at the knee joint
Legs (Hamstrings)	1. *Biceps femoris* 2. *Semitendinosus* 3. *Semimembranosus*	Flexion at the knee joint
Legs (Knees)	1. *Semitendinosus* 2. *Sartorius* 3. *Gracilis*	Medial rotation of the leg (tibia) when the knee is flexed
Legs (Calves)	*Gastrocnemius*	Plantar flexion at the ankle joint
Legs (Ankles)	1. Muscles of the *peroneus longus* and the *peroneus brevis*: • *Gastrocnemius* • *Soleus* • *Plantaris* • *Popliteus* • *Posterior tibialis* • *Flexor digitorum longus* • *Flexor hallucis longus* 2. *Anterior tibialis* 3. *Extensor digitorum longus* 4. *Extensor hallucis longus*	1. Plantar flexion at the ankle joint 2–4. Dorsiflexion at the ankle joint
Legs (Feet)	1. *Peroneus longus* 2. *Peroneus brevis* 3. *Anterior tibialis* 4. *Posterior tibialis*	1–2. Eversion at the foot 3–4. Inversion at the foot

Chart 2: Buttocks & Abdominals

Major Skeletal Muscles of the Body	Groups of Muscles That Form Each Skeletal Muscle	Primary Joint Motions
Buttocks (Glutei)	1. *Gluteus maximus*	1. Extension and lateral rotation at the Hip Joint
	2. *Gluteus medius*	2. Abduction at the Hip Joint
	3. *Gluteus minimus*	3. Abduction at the Hip Joint
Abdominals	1. *Rectus abdominis*	1. Flexion of the torso
	2. *External oblique*	2. Lateral rotation
	3. *Internal oblique*	3. Lateral rotation
	4. *Transverse abdominis*	4. Compresses the abdomen

Chart 3: Back

Major Skeletal Muscles of the Body	Groups of Muscles That Form Each Skeletal Muscle	Primary Joint Motions
Back	1. *Latissimus dorsi*	1. Extension, adduction, and medial rotation at the shoulder joint
	2. *Rhomboids (major and minor)*	2. Adduction and elevation of the scapula
	3. *Upper trapezius*	3. Elevation of the scapula
	4. *Middle trapezius*	4. Adduction of the scapula
	5. *Lower trapezius*	5. Depression of the scapula

Chart 4: Chest & Shoulders

Major Skeletal Muscles of the Body	Groups of Muscles That Form Each Skeletal Muscle	Primary Joint Motions
Chest	1. Pectoralis major	Flexion, adduction, and medial rotation at the shoulder joint
Shoulders (Deltoids)	1. Front deltoids	1. Flexion at the shoulder joint
	2. Middle deltoids	2. Abduction at the shoulder joint
	3. Rear deltoids	3. Lateral rotation at the shoulder joint
Shoulders (Rotator Cuff)	1. Supraspinatus	1. Abduction of the arm
	2. Infraspinatus	2. Lateral rotation of the arm
	3. Teres minor	3. Lateral rotation of the arm
	4. Subscapularis	4. Medial rotation of the arm

Chart 5: Biceps & Triceps

Major Skeletal Muscles of the Body	Groups of Muscles That Form Each Skeletal Muscle	Primary Joint Motions
Biceps	1. *Biceps Brachii*	1. Flexion at the elbow joint Flexion at the shoulder joint Supination of the forearm
	2. *Brachialis*	2. Flexion at the elbow joint
	3. *Brachioradialis*	3. Flexion at the elbow joint Pronation and supination of the forearm
Triceps	*Triceps brachii*	Extension at the elbow joint

Chart 6: Forearms & Wrist

Major Skeletal Muscles of the Body	Groups of Muscles That Form Each Skeletal Muscle	Primary Joint Motions
Forearms	*Pronator teres*	Pronation at the forearm (rotates so that the palm faces backward)
Wrist	1. *Flexor carpi radialis*	1. Wrist flexion Wrist abduction
	2. *Flexor carpi ulnaris*	2. Wrist flexion Wrist adduction
	3. *Extensor carpi radialis (longus and brevis)*	3. Wrist extension
	4. *Extensor carpi ulnaris*	4. Wrist extension Wrist adduction

1.1.11

Connective Tissue Types

- **Tendons**
  - **Aponeurosis**
- **Ligaments**
- **Fascia**
- **Cartilage**
  - *Hyaline cartilage*
  - *Fibrocartilage*
    - *Meniscus*
  - *Elastic cartilage*

Tendons
- Connective tissues that <u>attach muscle to bone</u>.
- Some skeletal muscles are attached to bone with a <u>broad, flat type of tendon known as *aponeurosis*</u>. A good example of aponeurosis is the wide, flat tendon insertion used by the abdominals.

Ligaments
- Connective tissues that <u>attach bone to bone</u>.

Fascia
- Connective tissues that <u>attach muscle to muscle</u>.

Cartilage
- A type of connective tissue that acts as an important structural component in many areas of the skeletal system.
- The most commonly referred to areas for cartilage are the joints.
- There are three main types of cartilage:

    1. *Hyaline cartilage*, the most abundant type of cartilage in the body, is found in most of the synovial joints, at the ends of bones.
        - This type of cartilage is a tough, smooth substance that provides a virtually frictionless surface within the joint.

    2. *Fibrocartilage* is a type of cartilage that is solid and very strong. It makes up the intervertebral discs between the bones of the spine.

        - *Meniscus* refers to the discs found in some of the synovial joints that are made of *fibrocartilage*. The *menisci* (the plural of *meniscus*) are cartilages that are used to divide the joint cavity into two separate cavities.
        - The *menisci* are especially important in weight-bearing joints such as the knee because they help to increase stability of the joint and absorb shock.
        - They also assist in nutrition of the joint by directing the flow of synovial fluid within the joint.
        - A common knee injury among athletes is the tearing of a *meniscus*, which is generally referred to as a *torn meniscus* or *torn cartilage*.

    3. *Elastic cartilage* is the flexible cartilage that is found in various parts of the body such as the outer ear and the epiglottis.

1.2
Stretching & Flexibility

1.2.1

Muscle Stretching vs. Muscle Contraction and Stabilization

Stretching is the elongation of muscle tissue and connective tissue, and it varies greatly from muscle contraction and stabilization.

Stretching
- When muscle fibers are lengthened to increase flexibility.

Contraction
- When muscle fibers contract to create a force that resists an opposing force. Depending on whether the muscles are contracting eccentrically or concentrically, a muscle may either lengthen or shorten during contraction.

Stabilization
- When muscle fibers of both the agonist muscle and the antagonist muscle (*muscle pairs*) contract with equal force to keep a joint from moving.

1.2.2

Flexibility of Joints

- **Range of Motion**
- **Static Flexibility**
- **Ballistic Flexibility**

- Flexibility describes the **range of motion** of a joint (the distance and direction a joint can move between the flexed position and the extended position).

- Flexibility can be improved by applying a force (e.g., a stretch or tension) to a body part by using proper technique in order to overcome the resistive forces from within the joint.

- **Static flexibility** describes the range of motion as it relates to a particular joint, and speed of movement is not an important consideration.

- **Ballistic (dynamic) flexibility** describes the resistance to motion as it relates to a particular joint, and speed of movement is an important consideration.

1.2.3

Flexibility of Connective Tissue

- **Elastic Property (or Elastic Elongation)**
- **Viscous Property (or Plastic Elongation Deformation)**

The connective tissues of the body combine two mechanical properties that function to accomplish flexibility:

Elastic Property
- Also known as *elastic elongation*, this is the ability of connective tissue to be elongated and then to recover after the tension has been removed.

Viscous Property
- Also known as *plastic elongation deformation*, this is when the deformation of the elongated connective tissue is permanent, or unrecoverable.

1.2.4

Types of Stretching

- **Static Stretch**
    - Passive
    - Active
- **Dynamic (Ballistic) Stretches**
- **Proprioceptive Neuromuscular Facilitation**

Stretching refers to the <u>elongation</u> of muscle tissue or connective tissue. Following are the most popular types of stretches:

Static Stretch
- <u>Application of a comfortable stretching force</u> to a muscle or muscle group, which is held for thirty seconds with absolutely no movement once the stretch position has been attained.
- This is the most common stretching technique. It is both highly effective and also the safest stretch technique.

- There are two types of static stretches:

    1. *Passive Static Stretch*
    With assistance from a trainer, your own body weight, or a device adds an external force to increase intensity. For example:
        - For a passive quadriceps stretch, a trainer will bend your knee while pushing the heel of your foot as close as possible to your buttocks.
        - The trainer will maintain the stretch for thirty seconds.
        - The connective tissue is the section of the quadriceps that is most affected by this stretch and where the stretch has greater permanence.

    2. *Active Static Stretch*
    Holding a body part in a stretched position with no assistance other than using the strength of agonist muscles. For example:
        - For an active hamstring stretch, stand on one leg and hold the opposite leg out directly in front of you, in an extended position, and without any assistance other than from your quadriceps.
        - The tension of the agonist muscles (quadriceps) in an active stretch helps to relax the antagonist muscles (hamstrings) that are being stretched.

Dynamic (Ballistic) Stretches
- These types of stretches are primarily used in athletic drills and use rapid, uncontrolled, bobbing or bouncing motions for short durations. They are designed to activate the stretch reflex.
- In these types of stretches, the use of continuous and exaggerated movements that simulate those of a person's sport or exercise results in improved flexibility for that sport. For example:
    - A runner using extra long strides to train for competition.
    - A basketball player jumping on and off of an exercise box (also referred to as *plyometrics*) to target flexibility in the hamstrings and lower back, muscle groups that are used in that sport.
- These short-duration, high-force exercises cause muscle spindle activity (a reaction that causes fibers in the muscle tissue to protect against too much stretch).
- This results in an increase in muscular reflex contraction to protect against this excessive stretch.
- When a muscle contracts (it becomes the agonist), and there is an opposite muscle that stretches (it becomes the antagonist), and it opposes the contraction.
- In short, the high forces of dynamic stretching exercises cause greater muscular contraction, and that is why there is greater muscle stretch.
- **Warning:** Ballistic stretching can be dangerous because there is a risk of tearing a muscle or connective tissue. Most therapists, doctors, and trainers consider ballistic stretching to be risky.

Proprioceptive Neuromuscular Facilitation (PNF)
- PNF is a method of stretching that is also referred to as the *contract/relax method*. This technique of stretching is designed to gain a greater degree of stretch in a muscle than conventional techniques by involving teamwork between a client and fitness professional.
- The client applies a maximum contraction, while at the same time the professional applies an equal resistance to the end of the client's limb. For example, the professional applies resistance to the foot when performing a hamstring stretch, and this resistance is applied at the end of the range of motion (the point where the leg is at or near the vertical position when the client is lying on his or her back).
- Remember, the teamwork component requires that the client must apply a maximum contraction at the same time. This method results in an isometric contraction and is held for a period of approximately six seconds. This is followed by the client's conscious relaxation of the involved muscle and the implementation of a maximum passive stretch by the professional.
- This procedure is repeated a few times, and it is believed that this technique accomplishes a superior stretch.

1.2.5

Neurophysiological Effects of Stretching

- **Myotatic Reflex**
    - **Golgi Tendon Organ (GTO)**
    - **Muscle Spindles**
- **Proprioceptors**

Myotatic Reflex
- The stretch reflex that is produced by neurophysiological responses in the body.
- The two neural receptors (sense organs) associated with the myotatic reflex are:

Golgi Tendon Organ (GTO)
- A sensory organ located in the tendons that, when stimulated by too much contractile force, will cause its related muscle or connective tissue to relax in order to protect against injury.

Muscle Spindles
- Fibers in the muscle tissue that protect against too much stretch, such as in ballistic stretching (rapid bouncing).
- When the muscle spindle is stimulated from ballistic stretching, it causes the involved muscle to contract as protection against this excessive stretch.
- Once this occurs, another rapid bounce or excessive stretch against the contracted muscle could cause serious damage to the muscle or its connective tissue.

Proprioceptors
- The components of muscles, tendons, and joints where <u>special nerve endings</u> detect any changes in movement, position, physical tension, or forces that occur to the body during an activity.
- These reactions enable the moving body part to gain a sense of relativity to its surroundings.

1.2.6

Safety Responses to Muscle Contraction & Muscle Stretching

- Reciprocal Innervation Inhibition
- Autogenic Inhibition

Reciprocal Innervation Inhibition
- Remember, when a muscle is contracted (the agonist muscle), there is another muscle that is stretching and opposing that action (the antagonist muscle) (see section 1.1.7).
- Reciprocal innervation inhibition refers to the body's protective reflex reaction to safeguard against muscle contraction, inhibiting the action of the antagonist muscle.
- For example, when the quadriceps is contracted, the action of the hamstring is inhibited as a protective reaction.
- Muscle spindles are the sensory organs responsible for this reflex reaction (see section 1.2.5).

Autogenic Inhibition
- Under normal conditions and up to a certain point, muscles will contract as a protective action against too much stretching.
- Autogenic inhibition refers to the body's protective reflex action against a stretch that is extreme enough to cause a rupture.
- This action causes the muscle to suddenly stop contracting and enables the muscles to relax.
- The Golgi tendon organ is the sensory organ responsible for this protective reflex reaction (see section 1.2.5).

1.3 Musculoskeletal Injuries and Conditions

1.3.1

Common Musculoskeletal Injuries and Conditions

- Sprains versus Strains
- Tendonitis
- Bursitis
- Dislocation
- Subluxation
- Hyperextension
- Concussion
- Low Back Pain
- Tennis Elbow
- Biceps Tendon Rupture
- Shoulder Impingement Syndrome
- Rotator Cuff Tear

Sprains versus Strains
- These two terms are often used inaccurately. Specifically, some people use the word *sprain* when the correct term would be *strain* and vice versa. So it is important to learn the difference:
    - **Sprain** refers to a ligament or joint capsule that has been overstretched or torn.
    - **Strain** refers to a muscle or tendon that has been overstretched or torn.

55

Tendonitis
- Inflammation of a tendon that results in pain and limited function to the affected area.
- It is extremely important to understand that tendonitis can possibly lead to a tendon rupture, so it is critical that you never ignore an inflamed tendon.
- Also, people who have had cortisone injections to treat tendonitis have a greater chance of it leading to a tendon rupture. Medical attention is recommended.

Bursitis
- Inflammation of the bursa, which results in pain to the affected area.
- The bursa is a fluid-filled sac that is covered by a synovial membrane. Inside the sac is a capillary layer of viscous fluid that acts as a cushion between the bones and tendons, or as a cushion for muscles around a joint, or both. The bursa reduces friction between the bones, which enhances free motion.
- Most frequently, bursitis occurs in the shoulders, elbows, hips, and knees. Medical attention is recommended.

Dislocation
- When a bone is separated from its normal position in the joint, such as a shoulder dislocation.

Subluxation
- A partial separation (dislocation) of a joint.

Hyperextension
- A high-risk position at a joint where the angle between the two involved bones is beyond the neutral position.
- An example of hyperextension at the shoulder joint would be doing the pull-down exercise behind the head. A safer method would be doing the pull-down exercise in front of the head where there would be no hyperextension at the shoulder joint.

Concussion
- A <u>sudden disturbance of electrical activity within the brain after a severe blow to the head, neck, or face,</u> which may result in permanent damage to the brain.
- The probability of seriousness increases for those who have had multiple concussions.
- A severe blow to another part of the body may also cause a concussion when the forces are powerful enough to be transmitted to the head.
- Concussions may or may not result in unconsciousness. If a person does become unconscious, it usually lasts only a few seconds.
- Accidents and sports are leading causes of concussions.
- Concussions are more likely to happen to football players, boxers, and anyone who participates in violent sports.
- Immediate medical assistance should be given to anyone who has suffered a concussion.
- The usual symptoms immediately following a concussion include confusion, dizziness, headache, seeing stars, feeling dazed, slurred speech, blurred vision, difficulty remembering, and vomiting.

Low Back Pain
- There are <u>many possible causes</u> for low back pain, including strains, sprains, ruptured disks, or disease. Consequently, we recommend that a physician diagnose all back pain.
- Sometimes a program of core exercises (abdominal muscle strength exercises) can relieve back pain. The abdominal muscle group can assist in supporting the torso, thus relieving some of the strain placed on the lower back.
- When an individual is in pain or spasm, the use of ice is a very effective way to relieve this condition. However, swift medical attention is recommended.

Tennis Elbow (Epicondylitis)
- Inflammation and pain at the elbow joint that is a result of overusing the forearm muscles.
- Epicondylitis typically occurs with people who play tennis or golf, lift weights, or participate in any other sport where excessive or improper use of the forearm can occur.
- The recommended treatment is to give the affected area partial or total rest and to treat with ice. Medical attention is recommended for this condition.
- Common sense and correct training practices should always be implemented for any sport in order to help prevent epicondylitis.

Biceps Tendon Rupture
- The bicep muscle has two separate tendons (the long head and the short head), which are located near the shoulder joint. When there is a rupture it usually occurs to the long-head tendon.
- One common cause is using too much weight during body building.
- Another common cause may be due to an accident where a powerful, external force is exerted on the bicep while it is in a contracted position.
- A biceps tendon rupture is a medical emergency and the individual should immediately be brought to a hospital emergency room.

Shoulder Impingement Syndrome
- Also known as a pinching injury, shoulder impingement is caused when the rotator cuff muscles and the bursa cannot pass smoothly through the *coracoacromial arch*, a narrow bony space that is located at the top of the shoulder.
- This restriction causes inflammation to the rotator cuff and bursa, which is then followed by pain and swelling. These painful conditions are referred to as rotator cuff tendinitis and bursitis, respectively, and cause pain when raising the arms above the head.
- Shoulder impingement is especially limiting for those who are weight lifters, swimmers, tennis players, baseball players, painters, and others who do work where raising the arms over the head is required.
- Medical attention is recommended.

Rotator Cuff Tear
- The rotator cuff is a group of <u>four muscles located at the shoulder</u>:
    1. *Supraspinatus*: responsible for <u>abduction</u> of the arm.
    2. *Infraspinatus*: responsible for <u>lateral rotation</u> of the arm.
    3. *Teres minor*: responsible for <u>lateral rotation</u> of the arm.
    4. *Subscapularis*: responsible for <u>medial rotation</u> of the arm.
- Certain diseases and injuries may cause tears to one or more of these muscles, resulting in pain and limited function.
- Medical attention is recommended.

1.3.2

Common Leg Injuries and Conditions

- Shin Splints
- Ankle Sprains
- Plantar Fasciitis
- Achilles Tendonitis and Rupture
- Chondromalacia Patella
- Patellofemoral Pain Syndrome
- Patellar Tendonitis (Jumpers Knee)
- Iliotibial Band Syndrome (ITB)
- Cartilage (Meniscus) Tears
- Anterior Cruciate Ligament (ACL) Tear

Shin Splints

- Any pain occurring to the front-inside area of the lower leg along the *tibia*, caused by inflammation to the attachment of the deep muscles in that area.
- Because diagnosis is sometimes challenging, and shin splints are sometimes thought to be stress fractures, or vice versa, it is important to understand two major differences:
    1. Shin splints affect muscles, the pain is not necessarily localized, and it can affect either a small area along the tibia or run the entire length of the tibia.
    2. Stress fractures affect bones, and the pain is localized (see section 2.2.2).
- Shin splints are a muscle overuse injury that usually results from the repetitive pounding effects of running, including intrinsic and/or extrinsic factors. When this activity is reduced or stopped, the pain will usually decrease.
- It is helpful to apply the methods outlined in the RICE procedure (see section 1.3.4), and treatment usually includes strengthening and flexibility exercises for the leg.
- If the pain continues, there is a possibility that the condition may instead be a stress fracture. Medical attention is recommended to diagnose and treat the problem.

Ankle Sprains

- The most common site of ankle sprains is to the outside of the ankle, although on rare occasions, it does happen to the inside of the ankle.
- The usual symptoms are swelling and an inability to walk on the affected foot. Within a couple of days, discoloration of the ankle usually appears.
- It is important to apply the methods outlined in the RICE procedure immediately after the injury to prevent additional swelling and further injury (see section 1.3.4). Medical attention is recommended.

Plantar Fasciitis
- Inflammation of the *plantar fascia*, which is the primary supportive soft tissue that comprises the sole of the foot.
- Plantar fasciitis results from recurring trauma that causes chronic inflammation to the plantar fascia.
- Common causes are running, improper training technique, always running in the same horizontal direction along a hill, and improperly fitting or worn-out footwear.
- It is also believed that high arches can make a person more likely to suffer from this condition.
- The best treatment is to eliminate the cause. Medical attention is recommended.

Achilles Tendonitis and Rupture
- The Achilles tendon is a powerful tendon that attaches both the *gastrocnemius* and the *soleus* muscles to the heel.
- There are a great variety of causes of inflammation or rupture, including sports involving jumping (e.g., basketball, volleyball, or aerobics) or footwear that is poorly cushioned or has stiff soles.
- If possible, eliminate the cause of inflammation to enable the tendon to heal. It is extremely important to understand that tendonitis can possibly lead to a tendon rupture. Therefore, it is critical that you never ignore an inflamed tendon.
- Also, people who have had cortisone injections to treat the inflammation have a greater predisposition to a tendon rupture. Medical attention is recommended.
- A ruptured Achilles tendon is a medical emergency and the individual should immediately be brought to a hospital emergency room.

Chondromalacia Patella
- Pain on the back of the patella (kneecap) due to the softening of cartilage there.
- The word *chondromalacia* specifically means "soft cartilage." In this condition, the articular cartilage gets soft and becomes diseased.
- For the purpose of making a diagnosis, it should be noted that pain around the kneecap does not necessarily indicate the condition known as chondromalacia patella. Medical attention is recommended.

Patellofemoral Pain Syndrome
- Pain around and under the patella (kneecap) due to a tracking problem.
- This painful condition is sometimes mistaken for chondromalacia patella.
- Tracking problems of the knee are often caused by a structural abnormality or some imbalance in the lower limb. In this situation, the patella does not have normal movement along the body groove that lies below the patella. The abnormal tracking is usually to the lateral side (outside).
- In addition to pain, symptoms include swelling and grinding. If swelling is present, it will be around and above the knee. To treat the pain and swelling, it is helpful to apply the methods outlined in the RICE procedure (see section 1.3.4).
- Common causes of this problem are squats or leg extensions with too much weight, improper form, and other exercises, including running, where intensity or duration is too excessive.
- Strengthening and flexibility exercises for the leg are excellent preventative measures.
- Other people may suffer from biomechanical problems such as muscle imbalances, which require professional help. Medical attention is recommended.

Patellar Tendonitis (Jumpers Knee)
- Inflammation of the patellar tendon, which extends from the bottom of the patella downward for approximately one to two inches.
- Inflammation of this tendon is usually caused by repetitive jumping activities, such as basketball, high jumping, volleyball, and certain aerobics.
- When the condition first develops, the pain is usually present only after the activity. If the condition worsens, the pain becomes more constant.
- The best overall treatment is cutting back or eliminating the particular type of activity that causes the problem.
- Strengthening and flexibility exercises for the leg are excellent preventative measures.
- It is extremely important to understand that tendonitis can possibly lead to a tendon rupture. Therefore, it is critical that you never ignore an inflamed tendon. Also, people who have had cortisone injections to treat the inflammation have a greater predisposition to a tendon rupture. Medical attention is recommended.

Iliotibial Band Syndrome (ITB)
- The *iliotibial band* is a thick structure of fascia that extends down across the lateral (outside) section of the knee.
- The most common cause of inflammation to the iliotibial band is frequent running on uneven ground, downhill running, or running along a sloped surface.
- The pain associated with this condition is usually felt just above the knee, and in more severe cases, the pain is felt up along the lateral thigh area.
- The best treatment is cutting back or eliminating the particular type of running that causes the inflammation. Medical attention is recommended.

Cartilage (Meniscus) Tears
- The medial and lateral cartilages (meniscus) are vital for stability and cushioning of the knee joint.
- There are many reasons why a cartilage can become torn, including injury, disease, and athletic activities such as weight lifting (particularly squatting), aerobic exercises, or running. In fact, any activity that subjects the knee to either prolonged stress or to excessive weight can cause a cartilage tear.
- Forces that cause the knee to bend or straighten too far also can result in a tear.
- The usual symptoms are pain, swelling, clicking, popping, locking, giving way, and crackling (*crepitus*).
- Meniscal tears usually require arthroscopic surgery. Continuing to exercise with a tear is not advisable. Medical attention is recommended.

Anterior Cruciate Ligament (ACL) Tears
- The ACL is located in the center of the knee and is vital for the stability of the joint.
- ACL tears usually occur in sports such as football and basketball as a result of a blow to the outside of the knee.
- ACL tears can also occur as a result of not landing properly after a jump or getting shoes caught in an irregularity of the playing surface.
- Diseases such as osteoarthritis can predispose the knee to an ACL tear.
- Symptoms include swelling, pain, popping, and instability at the knee joint.
- If the ACL sufferer wishes to continue exercising or participating in a sport, surgery is the likely course of action. Medical attention is recommended.

1.3.3

Overstretching (Stretch Weakness)

Stretch Weakness
- A condition that results when muscles have been overstretched for an extended period of time.
- The weakening effect on muscles creates a vulnerability to injury.
- It is important to use proper stretching technique and to understand that "more does not mean better."

1.3.4

Techniques Used to Treat Muscle Injury (RICE)

Many <u>muscular injures</u> can benefit by the immediate use of RICE techniques, but *always consult a physician before using these techniques.*

The acronym "RICE" stands for:
1. Rest
2. Ice
3. Compression
4. Elevation

Rest
- Avoid activities that affect the injured area.
- Rest is required in order to allow damaged tissue an opportunity to heal.

Ice
- Often the first treatment following an injury, ice should be applied for a period of <u>twenty to thirty minutes at a time, or as medically recommended.</u> Be sure to use a layer of insulation, such as a towel, to prevent damage to the skin.
- Depending on the severity of the injury, the application of ice should be continued between <u>four to eight times per day, or as medically recommended.</u>
- The benefits of using ice on an injury include reducing inflammation and swelling, which promotes more rapid healing.
- Caution: Do not apply ice to a numb area.

Compression
- The use of an elastic bandage is a highly effective way to compress an injured area in order to prevent or reduce swelling by forcing fluids back into the body, which in turn promotes more rapid healing.

Elevation
- Once the first three measures have been taken, raising the injured part of the body slightly above the heart enables gravity to assist in the reduction of swelling as well.

1.3.5

Muscular System Testing Devices

- Electromyogram (EMG)
- Dynamometer
- Inclinometer
- Goniometer

Electromyogram (EMG)
- When muscles are active, they produce an electrical current. This current is usually proportional to the level of the muscle activity.
- <u>EMGs are used to detect abnormal electrical activity of muscles</u> due to health conditions or injury. Examples include damage to nerves in the arms and legs (peripheral nerve damage), inflammation of muscles, disk herniation, muscular dystrophy, myasthenia gravis, amyotrophic lateral sclerosis (ALS), and others.

Dynamometer
- Tests for muscle forces during exercise (i.e., the force exerted by a muscle).
- A typical example would be to measure the force exerted by the quadriceps muscle during a leg extension exercise.

Inclinometer
- An angle gauge used for testing a person's range of motion (the distance and direction a joint can move between the flexed position and the extended position).
- Medical assessments pertaining to health conditions, post operative limitations, and injury are the primary reasons for performing this test.

Goniometer
- Another type of angle gauge used for testing a person's range of motion.

CHAPTER 2

The Skeletal System

2.1 Anatomy of the Skeletal System ································· 73
    2.1.1   Skeletal Categories and Functions ························· 75
    2.1.2   Standard Anatomical Position ···························· 76
    2.1.3   Axial Skeleton ··· 78
    2.1.4   Appendicular Skeleton ·································· 79
    2.1.5   Bones of the Skull ····································· 80
    2.1.6   Bones of the Vertebral Column ·························· 82
    2.1.7   Joints ·· 84
    2.1.8   Three Primary Joints Types ····························· 85
    2.1.9   Anatomical Planes ····································· 86
    2.1.10 Synovial Joint Motions ································· 88
    2.1.11 Mechanics of Synovial Joints ··························· 91

2.2 Skeletal System Injuries and Conditions ························ 93
    2.2.1   Arthritis ·· 95
    2.2.2   Stress Fracture ·· 99
    2.2.3   Posture Abnormalities ································· 100
    2.2.4   Cortisone for Pain Relief ······························· 101

2.1 Anatomy of the Skeletal System

2.1.1

Skeletal Categories and Functions

- The skeletal system of the human body is comprised of <u>206 bones</u>.
- These bones can be divided into <u>two categories</u>:

    1. **Axial Skeleton**: Eighty bones that form the head, neck, and trunk.

    2. **Appendicular Skeleton**: One hundred twenty-six bones that comprise the extremities.

- The skeletal system provides <u>five major functions</u> for the body:

    1. Protection for many vital organs, including the heart, brain, and spinal cord.
    2. Support that enables the body to sustain its form and its erect posture.
    3. Structure comprised of levers that have muscles attached to them to create movement.
    4. Production of red blood cells, certain types of white blood cells, and blood platelets (which all occurs in the red marrow of the bones).
    5. Storage area for calcium, phosphorus, potassium, sodium, and certain other minerals.

2.1.2

Standard Anatomical Position

- **Standard Anatomical Position** a term used as reference to describe the following three positions:

    1. **Body** *standing erect*
    2. **Feet** *facing forward*
    3. **Palms** *facing forward*

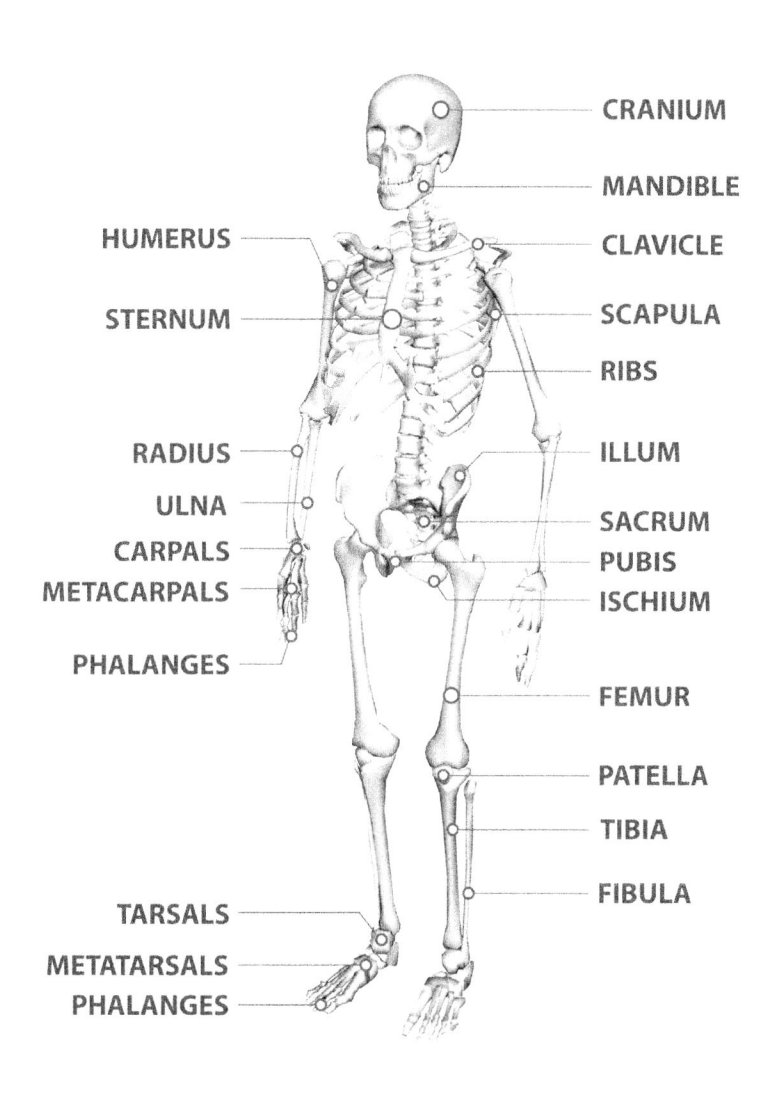

CRANIUM
MANDIBLE
HUMERUS
CLAVICLE
STERNUM
SCAPULA
RIBS
RADIUS
ILLUM
ULNA
SACRUM
CARPALS
PUBIS
METACARPALS
ISCHIUM
PHALANGES
FEMUR
PATELLA
TIBIA
FIBULA
TARSALS
METATARSALS
PHALANGES

- The illustration above shows twenty-three of the 206 bones of the human body.

2.1.3

Axial Skeleton

Eighty bones make up the head, neck, and trunk:

- Cranium .... 8 bones
- Face .... 14 bones
- Hyoid Bone .... 1 bone (located in the neck)
- Ears .... 6 bones (auditory ossicles)
- Vertebral Column .... 26 movable bones
- Sternum .... 1 bone
- Ribs .... 24 bones

2.1.4

Appendicular Skeleton

One hundred twenty-six bones make up the legs and arms:

- Phalanges (upper) .... 28 bones
- Phalanges (lower) .... 28 bones
- Metatarsals .... 10 bones
- Tarsals .... 14 bones
- Patella .... 2 bones
- Tibia .... 2 bones
- Fibula .... 2 bones
- Femur .... 2 bones
- Hip and Pelvis .... 2 bones
- Clavicle .... 2 bones
- Scapula .... 2 bones
- Metacarpals .... 10 bones
- Carpals .... 16 bones
- Radius .... 2 bones
- Ulna .... 2 bones
- Humerus .... 2 bones

2.1.5

Bones of the Skull

- **Cranium**
- **Face**
- **Ears**

Twenty-eight bones make up the cranium, face, and ears:

Cranium
- Eight bones form the cranium, which surrounds the brain:
    - One frontal bone
    - Two temporal bones
    - Two parietal bones
    - One occipital bone
    - One ethmoid bone
    - One sphenoid bone

Face
- Fourteen bones form the cheek, jaw, and nasal cavity:

    - Two maxilla bones
    - Two palatine bones
    - Two zygomatic bones
    - Two lacrimal bones
    - Two nasal bones
    - One vomer bone
    - Two inferior nasal concha bones
    - One mandible (jaw bone)

Ears*
- Each is made up of three bones:

    - One malleus (hammer) per ear
    - One incus (anvil) per ear
    - One stapes (stirrup) per ear

---

* Technically, the ear bones are not considered part of either the axial skeleton or the appendicular skeleton. However, they are sometimes associated with the axial skeleton. The fact is, they are just part of the ear.

2.1.6

Bones of the Vertebral Column

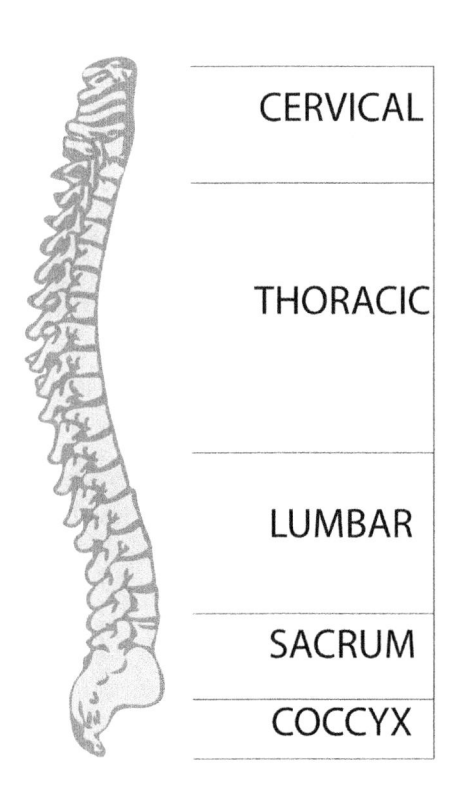

CERVICAL

THORACIC

LUMBAR

SACRUM

COCCYX

Vertebral Column
- Protects the spinal cord from injury.
- Encloses the spinal cord and the fluid surrounding it.
- Comprised of twenty-six bones, as follows:

    - **Seven cervical vertebrae** in the neck
    - **Twelve thoracic vertebrae** at the back wall of the chest
    - **Five lumbar vertebrae** at the inward curve of the small of the lower back
    - **One sacrum** comprised of five fused vertebrae between the hip bones
    - **One coccyx** comprised of four fused vertebrae at the lower tip of the vertebral column

2.1.7

Joints

- **Ligaments**
- **Joint Cavity**
- **Synovial Fluid**
- **Bursa**

Joints
- The points of contact or connection between bones, and between bones and cartilage.
- Also called <u>articulations.</u>

Ligaments
- The dense fibrous strands of connective tissue that link bones to bones and maintain the stability and integrity of all joints.

Joint Cavity
- The space between the connected bones.

Synovial Fluid
- The viscous, thick, lubricating fluid located within the joints of the body.
- Synovial fluid also provides nutrition to the cartilage within the joint.
- Sometimes when overuse or an acute injury occurs to a joint, the synovial membrane will produce an excess of synovial fluid. This, in turn, produces swelling and increases pain at the joint, particularly when movement occurs.

Bursa
- The sac that is located around a joint that reduces friction between bones and ligaments by secreting a lubricating fluid.

2.1.8

Three Primary Joints Types

- **Fibrous Joints**
- **Cartilaginous Joints**
- **Synovial Joints**

Major characteristics that define the three primary joint types are:
- The existence or nonexistence of a joint cavity.
- The type of connective tissue that holds a joint together.
- Types of motion the joint is capable of.

Fibrous Joints (Syndesmoses)
- Do not have a joint cavity but are held together by ligaments.
- Little or no motion occurs at these joints.
- Locations of this joint are in the skull and between the radius and ulna.

Cartilaginous Joints (Synchondroses)
- Do not have a joint cavity, and cartilage unites the bones.
- Little or no motion occurs at these joints.
- Locations of these joints are in the spinal cord and the connection between the ribs and the sternum.

Synovial Joints (Diarthroses)
- Have a joint cavity and are surrounded by fibrous connective tissue.
- Synovial is the largest functional category of joints and many different types of motions occur at their various locations throughout the body, including the knee, shoulder, elbow, and ankle.

2.1.9

Anatomical Planes

There are three primary planes:

1. **Sagittal Plane (Lateral Plane)**
   - An imaginary <u>vertical line</u> that divides the body or a body part into right and left sections.

2. **Frontal Plane (Coronal Plane)**
   - An imaginary <u>vertical line</u> that divides the body or a body part into anterior (front) and posterior (back) sections. The sagittal plane and the frontal plane bisect each other at right angles.

3. **Transverse Plane (Axial Plane)**
   - An imaginary <u>horizontal line</u> that divides the body or a body part into superior (upper) and inferior (lower) sections.

SPEED LEARNING FOR ANATOMY

Sagittal plane — Coronal plane *Frontal*

Transverse plane *Horizontal*

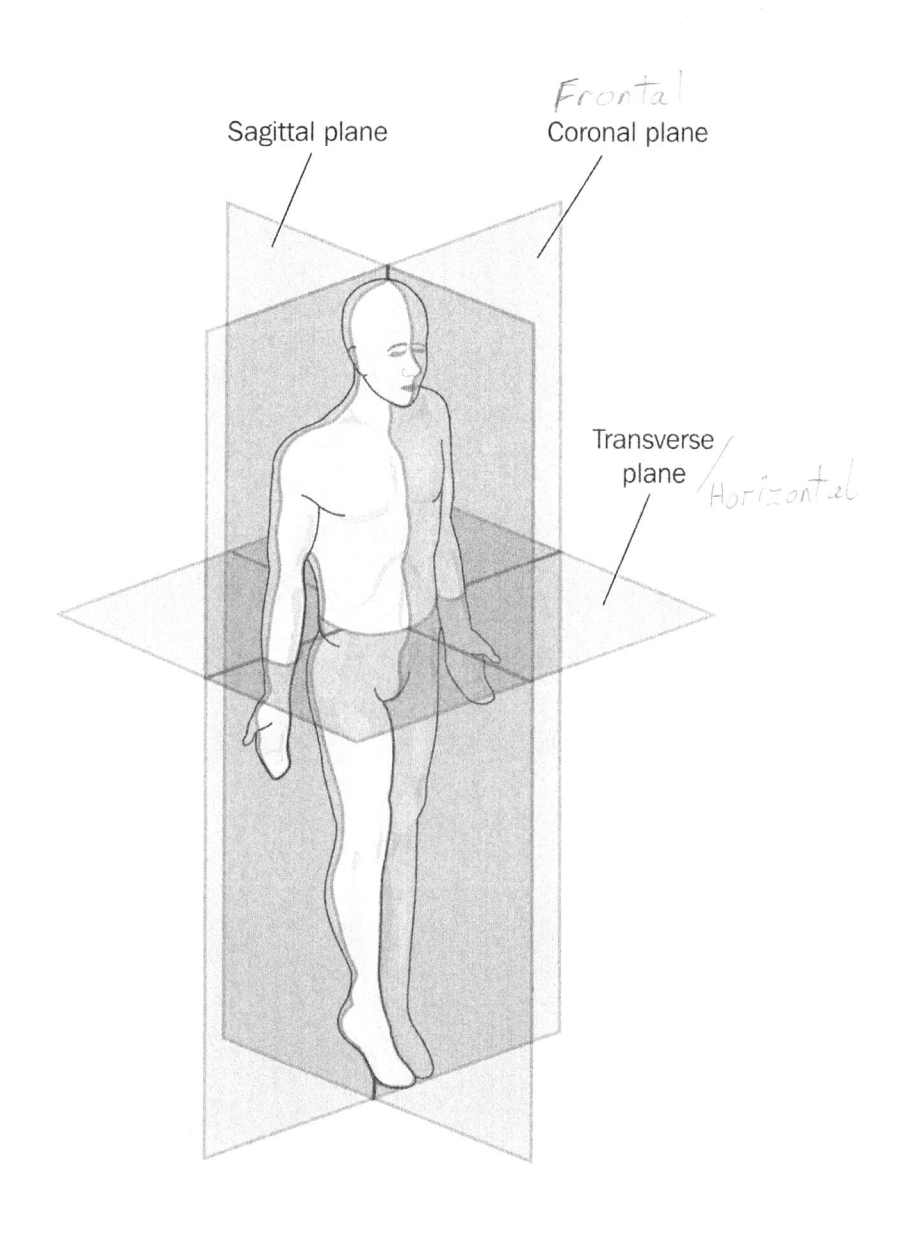

2.1.10

Synovial Joint Motions

- Flexion
- Extension
- Adduction
- Abduction
- Horizontal Flexion
- Horizontal Extension
- Elevation
- Depression
- Rotary Motion

- Rotation
- Inversion
- Eversion
- Plantar Flexion
- Dorsiflexion
- Pronation
- Supination
- Circumduction
- Opposition

Flexion creates motion on a *Sagittal Plane*
- **Action** brings two connected body parts closer together, like bending an elbow during the positive phase of a biceps curl. It is the ***opposite* of extension**.

Extension creates motion on a *Sagittal Plane*
- **Action** moves two connected body parts toward a straight line, like straightening the elbow during the negative phase of a biceps curl. It is the ***opposite* of flexion**.

Adduction creates motion on a *Frontal Plane*
- **Action** moves a body part ***toward* the midline** of the body.

Abduction creates motion on a *Frontal Plane*
- **Action** moves a body part *away* from the midline of the body.

Horizontal Flexion creates motion on a *Transverse Plane*
- **Action** as an example, if an arm starts off in a ninety-degree abducted position, the humerus is then flexed in *toward* the midline of the body.

Horizontal Extension creates motion on a *Transverse Plane*
- **Action** as an example, if an arm starts off in the adducted position, the humerus is extended *away* from the midline of the body out toward a ninety-degree abducted position.

Elevation creates motion on a *Frontal Plane*
- **Action** the scapula moves upward and away from the ribcage. Muscles involved are the upper trapezius, rhomboids, and the levator scapulae. Elevation applies only to motions where the shoulder is raised, whether by exercising or any other reason.

Depression creates motion on a *Frontal Plane*
- **Action** the scapula moves downward and toward the ribcage. Muscles involved are the lower trapezius, and the lower serratus anterior. Depression applies only to motions where the shoulder is lowered, whether by exercising or any other reason.

Rotary Motion creates motion on a *Transverse Plane*
- **Action** moving a body part around a nonmoving point. For example, turning your head right or left while keeping your trunk still.

Rotation creates motion on a *Transverse Plane*
- **Action** the inward (medial) or outward (lateral) turning of a body part around a bone that is fixed in a vertical position. For example, turning your upper body to the right or to the left while your feet remain stationary on the floor.

Inversion creates motion on a *Transverse Plane*
- **Action** the *inward* movement of the sole of the foot so that the sole faces *toward* the opposite foot. An anatomical term that only applies to the feet.

Eversion creates motion on a *Transverse Plane*
- **Action** the *outward* movement of the sole of the foot so that the sole faces *away* from the opposite foot. An anatomical term that only applies to the feet.

Plantar Flexion creates motion on a *Sagittal Plane*
- **Action** an ankle joint motion that moves the toes to a pointing *downward* position. An anatomical term that *only* applies to the feet.

Dorsiflexion creates motion on a *Sagittal Plane*
- **Action** an ankle joint motion that moves the toes to a pointing *upward* position. An anatomical term that *only* applies to the feet.

Pronation creates motion on a *Transverse Plane*
- **Action** when the forearm is positioned with the palm facing *downward or backward*. An anatomical term that *only* applies to the wrist.

Supination creates motion on a *Transverse Plane*
- **Action** when the forearm is positioned with the palm facing *upward or forward*. An anatomical term that *only* applies to the wrist.

Circumduction creates motion on a *Multiplanar Plane*
- **Action** a *circular movement* **similar to rotation**; particularly applicable to the shoulder and hip joints. This circular movement requires flexion, abduction, extension, and adduction all in sequential combination.

Opposition creates motion on a *Multiplanar Plane*
- **Action** in humans, it is the *unique movement of the thumb*. Opposition allows the hand to perform such actions as grabbing, squeezing, or holding an object.

2.1.11

Mechanics of Synovial Joints

Joint Type	Joint Location (Examples)	Movement
Hinge Joint	Knee Elbow Ankle	Movement is back and forth
Ball & Socket Joint	Hip Shoulder	Movement in all directions
Pivot Joint (Swivel Joint)	Neck	Movement is rotational
Gliding Joint (Planar Joint)	In the Carpal bones of the hand, and in the Tarsal bones of the feet	Movement is side to side, and up and down
Saddle Joint	Thumb	Movement in a wide range
Ellipsiod Joint (Condyloid Joint)	Wrist	Movement is side to side, and up and down

2.2 Skeletal System Injuries and Conditions

2.2.1

Arthritis

- **Rheumatoid Arthritis**
- **Osteoarthritis**
- **Ankylosing Spondylitis**
- **Seronegative Arthritis**
- **Still's Disease**
- **Infective Arthritis**
- **Gout**

Arthritis
- Inflammation of one or more joints.
- Symptoms include:
    - Joint pain (*arthralgia*)
    - Swelling
    - Stiffness
    - Redness in and around the affected area
    - Grating or grinding sound in a joint (*crepitus*)

JUSTINA C. BACHSTEINER PHD

Osteoarthritis and Normal Joint Anatomy

NORMAL JOINT

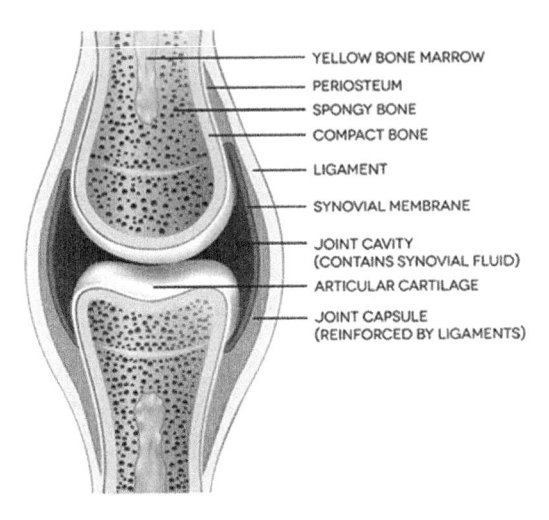

- YELLOW BONE MARROW
- PERIOSTEUM
- SPONGY BONE
- COMPACT BONE
- LIGAMENT
- SYNOVIAL MEMBRANE
- JOINT CAVITY (CONTAINS SYNOVIAL FLUID)
- ARTICULAR CARTILAGE
- JOINT CAPSULE (REINFORCED BY LIGAMENTS)

OSTEOARTHRITIS

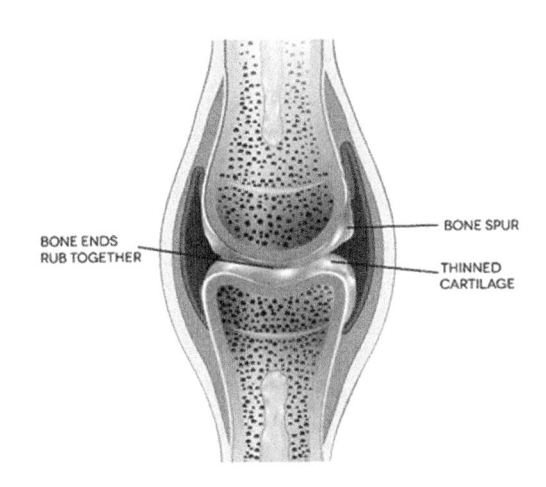

- BONE ENDS RUB TOGETHER
- BONE SPUR
- THINNED CARTILAGE

Some of the more common forms of arthritis are as follows:

Rheumatoid Arthritis
- An autoimmune disease (wherein the body's own immune system attacks the body's own tissues) that results in inflammation, pain, stiffness, swelling, and redness in the diseased joint.
- In severe cases the fingers, wrists, and/or toes become deformed.

Osteoarthritis
- Characterized mainly by the degeneration of the cartilage that lines and protects the joints of the body and outgrowths of new bone called osteophytes, particularly along the perimeter of the affected joint surface.
- These conditions result in inflammation, pain, stiffness, swelling, and redness in the diseased joint.

Ankylosing Spondylitis
- A type of arthritis that causes inflammation to the joints and ligaments to the spine.
- This causes pain and stiffness usually beginning in the lower back or buttocks area.
- Progression of this condition may also affect the upper spine, chest and neck.
- Eventually, vertebrae may connect to each other (fuse), resulting in a rigid and inflexible spine.
- As this disease progresses further, knee, hip and shoulder joints may also become affected.
- Ankylosing spondylitis is a *systemic disease*, and that means it may affect any number of organs and tissues, or affect the entire body.

Seronegative Arthritis
- May be related to certain skin disorders, such as psoriasis, and certain inflammatory intestinal disorders, such Crohn's disease.

Still's Disease
- A type of arthritis that affects children, usually under the age of four.

Infective Arthritis
- Inflammation of a joint as a result of an infected wound that is close to the joint or from an infection in the blood stream.
- Infective arthritis can cause a <u>dangerous condition</u> where there is the presence of bacteria or their toxins in the blood or tissues (*sepsis*), as well as be pus producing (*pyogenic*).

Gout
- Caused by an accumulation of uric acid in the joints.
- The uric acid build-up occurs in the form of crystals that creates joint inflammation.

2.2.2

Stress Fracture

- A limited type of <u>bone fracture</u> resulting from overuse.
- The most common occurrences are in the foot or the lower leg and are characterized by an aching pain that is <u>usually</u> <u>localized</u>.
- Continued stress on the affected bone could result in a complete fracture. Medical attention is recommended.
- Long-distance runners are most affected by this condition.
- Compare to shin splints in section 1.3.2.

2.2.3

Posture Abnormalities

- **Lordosis**
- **Kyphosis**
- **Scoliosis**

There are three classic abnormalities in posture:

Lordosis
- An increase in the normal forward curvature of the lumbar spine.
- The result is often a posture with a protruding abdomen and buttocks, rounded shoulders, and forward head.

Kyphosis
- An increase in the normal backward curvature of the thoracic spine.
- The result is often a posture with rounded shoulders, sunken chest, and a forward-downward head position.
- This abnormal head position is compensated for by an exaggerated tilt of the neck toward the rear of the body, referred to as hyperextension of the neck.

Scoliosis
- An abnormal curvature of the spine, commonly in the thoracic area.
- There are usually two abnormal curves, one to the right of the spine and the other to the left of the spine, or vice versa.
- These opposing curves tend to compensate for each other.

2.2.4

Cortisone for Pain Relief

- **Cortisone** is a popular steroid medication that is commonly injected into muscles, joints, and connective tissue to relieve pain by reducing inflammation.

- Too many cortisone injections may cause tissue damage, and occasionally, cause tendon rupture.

- Physical therapy is believed to be more effective than the use of cortisone for rehabilitating an injury. However, it is not always possible as the first step because the pain is too strong.

- Therefore, the temporary relief of cortisone can enable a patient to facilitate treatment by reducing or eliminating inflammation and pain, and rehabilitate an injury faster.

- The benefit of a cortisone injection should be weighed carefully against the risks before being used.

CHAPTER 3

The Digestive System

3.1 Anatomy of the Digestive System ·····································105
    3.1.1   Gastrointestinal Tract ··107
    3.1.2   Small Intestine ··110
    3.1.3   Large Intestine ··112
    3.1.4   Additional Digestive System Components ················113

3.2 Digestive System Injuries and Conditions ······················117
    3.2.1   Hernia ···119
    3.2.2   Peptic Ulcer ··121
    3.2.3   Irritable Bowel Syndrome (IBS) ·····························122
    3.2.4   Hemorrhoids ··124
    3.2.5   Crohn's Disease ···126
    3.2.6   Acid Reflux ···129

3.1 Anatomy of the Digestive System

3.1.1

Gastrointestinal Tract

- **Gastrointestinal (GI)** refers to the stomach and intestines, specifically the large, muscular tube that extends from the mouth to the anus, where the movement of muscles, along with the release of hormones and enzymes, allows for the digestion of food.

- Also called the *alimentary canal* or *digestive tract*.

- The GI tract is conventionally divided into upper and lower parts, with associated accessory organs.

Upper GI Tract
- This is where ingestion and the first phase of digestion occur and includes the following:
    - **Mouth** (see section 3.1.4)
    - **Pharynx** (see section 3.1.4)
    - **Esophagus**
    - **Stomach**

Human Gastrointestinal Tract

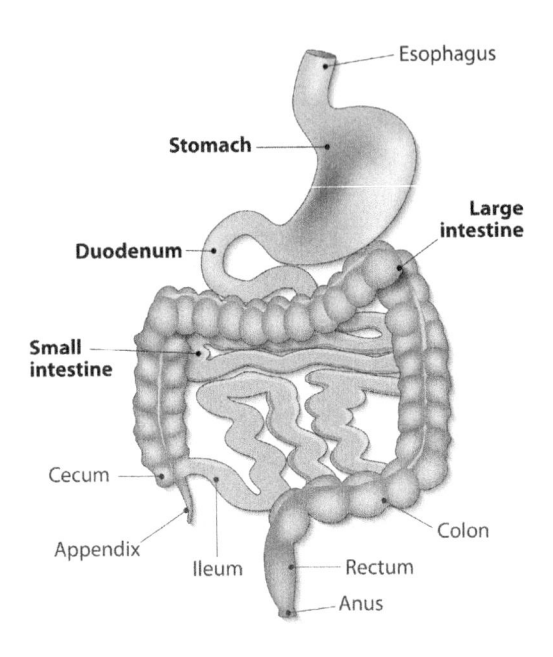

Esophagus
- The hollow tube that receives food from the pharynx (throat).
- Its purpose is to push this food to your stomach by a series of muscular contractions called *peristalsis*.

Stomach
- A large, sac-like organ where food is digested, the stomach receives food from the esophagus, which is connected at its upper segment.
- The stomach then sends the digested food out to the small intestine, which is connected at its lower segment.

Lower GI Tract
- Its primary function is the absorption of leftover water from the waste products of digestion, where it then compacts the remaining waste into feces for elimination.
- Lower GI tract components include the following:

Small Intestine
- Duodenum
- Jejunum
- Ileum

Large Intestine
- Cecum
- Appendix
- Colon
- Rectum
- Anus

3.1.2

Small Intestine

- Primarily responsible for the digestion of food and the absorption of food nutrients into the bloodstream.

- There are intestinal glands that are located in the lining of the small intestine that are responsible for secreting intestinal juices that aid in the digestive process.

- The three main sections of the small intestine are the following:

    1. **Duodenum**
        - The first part of the small intestine that connects to the stomach.
        - Helps to further digest food coming from the stomach.
        - Absorbs nutrients (vitamins, minerals, carbohydrates, fats, proteins) and water from food so they can be used by the body.

    2. **Jejunum** *(not shown in illustration)*
        - The middle part of the small intestine between the duodenum and the ileum.
        - Helps to further digest food coming from the duodenum.
        - Absorbs nutrients (vitamins, minerals, carbohydrates, fats, proteins) and water from food so they can be used by the body.

3. **Ileum**
    - <u>The last part of the small intestine</u> that connects to the first part of the large intestine.
    - Helps to further digest food coming from the stomach and other parts of the small intestine.
    - Absorbs nutrients (vitamins, minerals, carbohydrates, fats, proteins) and water from food so they can be used by the body, and delivers anything remaining to the large intestine.

3.1.3

Large Intestine

- The primary purpose of the large intestine is the removal of digestive waste products called feces.

- The four main sections of the large intestine are the following:

    1. **Cecum**
        - The beginning section of the large intestine.
        - Receives fecal material from the final section of the small intestine, the ileum.
        - Includes the *appendix*, a small, fingerlike pouch that sticks out from the cecum.

    2. **Colon**
        - A six-foot-long tubular section that connects the cecum to the rectum.
        - Primary purpose is to remove water from digested food that then results in the conversion to solid waste called stool.
        - Stool then travels through the colon into the rectum.

    3. **Rectum**
        - This is the last six to eight inches of the large intestine where stool is stored before it is evacuated from the anus.

    4. **Anus**
        - The opening of the rectum through which the stool is expelled from the body.

3.1.4

Additional Digestive System Components

- Mouth
- Saliva
- Salivary Glands
- Ptyalin
- Teeth
- Pharynx
- Chyme

- Gastric Juices
- Enzymes
- Pancreas
- Liver
- Gall Bladder

The digestive system <u>converts the food you eat into nutrients</u> that are used by the body for energy, repairing cells, and growth.

Mouth
- Begins the initial breakdown of food through chewing and aids in digestion by releasing saliva.

Saliva
- A digestive juice that is 99.5 percent water located in the mouth and manufactured by the salivary glands.
- The remaining 0.5 percent contains an enzyme known as *ptyalin* (see below).
- Also moistens the mouth to help a person chew, swallow food, and control bacteria that could cause mouth infection and tooth decay.

Salivary Glands
- There are three pairs of salivary glands in the mouth that produce saliva:
    1. *Parotid glands*: located in the mouth and in front of the ear
    2. *Submandibular glands*: located in the mouth and under the jaw
    3. *Sublingual glands*: located under the tongue, on the floor of the mouth

Ptyalin
- An enzyme found in the saliva that is used in the digestive process to break down the starches and glycogens that you put into your mouth.
- Once the starches and glycogens are covered with your saliva, they are broken down into maltose and glucose, which are simple sugars that can be used more readily by the body.

Teeth
- Primary function is to chew (masticate) and to mix food with saliva.
- Normally there are thirty-two permanent teeth in the adult mouth.

Pharynx (Throat)
- Receives broken-down food particles from the mouth.
- It is an organ of the respiratory system as well.

Chyme
- Partially digested food and the digestive secretions that are formed in the stomach and intestine during digestion.

Gastric Juices
- Digestive fluids secreted from glands located in the stomach.

Enzymes
- Organic compounds that are composed mostly of proteins and used in the process of digestion, enzymes act as <u>catalysts</u> because they produce changes in chemical reactions.
- These chemical reactions produce a series of chemical breakdowns to the body's complex compounds that results in the production of simpler substances, and the end result is the production of energy for the body's needs.

Pancreas
- A gland that is located behind and beneath the stomach, the pancreas has a duct portion that secretes a digestive juice known as pancreatic juice.
- The ductless portion of the pancreas is known as the *Islets of Langerhans* (also called the *Islands of Langerhans*), which produces insulin (a hormone that controls the proper levels of glucose within the cells of the body).

Liver
- The largest internal organ in the body that has several functions.
- Absorbs nutrients and oxygen from the blood.
- Regulates amino-acid levels in the blood.
- Regulates glucose levels in the blood.
- Produces important proteins, including *albumin*.
- Produces substances that contribute to the process of blood clotting (*co-agulation*) when bleeding occurs.
- Helps to break down and remove toxic substances and drugs from the blood.
- Is responsible for the production of bile, which removes waste from the liver and helps it to breakdown and absorb fats in the small intestine.
- Stores sugar in the form of glycogen.

Gall Bladder
- A sac that is attached to the liver, the gall bladder is used to store the bile that the liver produces.
- When digestion is required, the gall bladder releases the stored bile into the small intestine where it helps in the breakdown and absorption of fats.

3.2 Digestive System Injuries and Conditions

3.2.1

Hernia

- **Inguinal Hernia**
- **Umbilical Hernia**
- **Femoral Hernia**
- **Hiatal Hernia**

- **Hernia** is a condition that occurs when an organ or fatty tissue protrudes, squeezes, pushes, or passes through muscle tissue.
- There are several types of hernias, and they are classified by the body location where they occur.
- The following are four of the most common types.

Inguinal Hernia
- When contents of the abdomen, usually fat or part of the small intestine, bulge through a weak area in the lower abdominal wall, also called the inguinal or groin region.
- Two types of inguinal hernias are as follows:
    1. *Indirect inguinal hernias*: Caused by a defect in the abdominal wall that is congenital—or present at birth.
    2. *Direct inguinal hernias*: Usually occur only in adult males and are caused by a weakness in the muscles of the abdominal wall that develops over time.

Umbilical Hernia
- When part of the small intestine bulges out through the abdominal wall near the belly button or navel.

Femoral Hernia
- When the intestine protrudes through the lower abdomen in the area near the upper thigh.
- This condition is more common in women, particularly those who are obese or pregnant.

Hiatal Hernia
- When the opening of the diaphragm lets the upper part of the stomach move up into the chest, which lowers the pressure in the esophageal sphincter.

3.2.2

Peptic Ulcer

- A sore on the lining of your stomach or duodenum.

- Rarely, a peptic ulcer may develop just above the stomach in the esophagus. Doctors call this type of peptic ulcer an esophageal ulcer.

- Causes of peptic ulcers include:
    - Long-term use of nonsteroidal anti-inflammatory drugs (NSAIDs), such as aspirin and ibuprofen.
    - An infection with the bacteria *Helicobacter pylori*.
    - Rare cancerous and noncancerous tumors in the stomach, duodenum, or pancreas—known as Zollinger-Ellison syndrome.

3.2.3

Irritable Bowel Syndrome (IBS)

- A group of symptoms—including pain or discomfort in your abdomen and changes in your bowel movement patterns—that occur together.
- Doctors call IBS a functional gastrointestinal (GI) disorder.
- Functional GI disorders happen when your GI tract behaves in an abnormal way without evidence of damage due to a disease.
- In the past, doctors called IBS many other names, including *colitis, mucous colitis, spastic colon, nervous colon,* and *spastic bowel.*
- Experts changed the name to IBS to reflect the understanding that the disorder has both physical and mental causes and isn't a product of a person's imagination.
- Doctors often classify IBS into one of four types based on stool consistency.
- Differentiating the types is important because it will affect the types of treatment that are most likely to improve symptoms.

    1. **IBS with constipation, or IBS-C**
        - Hard or lumpy stools at least 25 percent of the time.
        - Loose or watery stools less than 25 percent of the time.

    2. **IBS with diarrhea, or IBS-D**
        - Loose or watery stools at least 25 percent of the time.
        - Hard or lumpy stools less than 25 percent of the time.

3. **Mixed IBS, or IBS-M**
   - Hard or lumpy stools at least 25 percent of the time.
   - Loose or watery stools at least 25 percent of the time.

4. **Unsubtyped IBS, or IBS-U**
   - Hard or lumpy stools less than 25 percent of the time.
   - Loose or watery stools less than 25 percent of the time.

3.2.4

Hemorrhoids

- Also called *piles*, hemorrhoids are swollen and inflamed veins around your anus or in your lower rectum.

- The <u>two types of hemorrhoids</u> are:
    - *External hemorrhoids*, which form under the skin around the anus.
    - *Internal hemorrhoids*, which form in the lining of the anus and lower rectum.

- Hemorrhoids are common in both men and women, and affect about one in twenty Americans.

- About half of adults older than age fifty have hemorrhoids.

- <u>High-risk triggers for hemorrhoids include the following</u>:
    - Straining during bowel movements
    - Sitting on the toilet for long periods of time
    - Having chronic constipation or diarrhea
    - Eating foods that are low in fiber
    - Pregnancy
    - Lifting heavy objects

- Complications of hemorrhoids can include the following:
    - Blood clots in an external hemorrhoid
    - Skin tags—extra skin left behind when a blood clot in an external hemorrhoid dissolves
    - Infection of a sore on an external hemorrhoid
    - Strangulated hemorrhoid—when the muscles around the anus cut off the blood supply to an internal hemorrhoid that has fallen through the anal opening.

3.2.5

Crohn's Disease

- A chronic disease that causes inflammation and irritation in your digestive tract.

- Most commonly, Crohn's affects the small intestine and the beginning of the large intestine. However, the disease can affect any part of the digestive tract, from mouth to anus.

- Crohn's disease is an inflammatory bowel disease (IBD).

- *Ulcerative colitis* and *microscopic colitis* are other common types of IBD.

- Crohn's disease most often begins gradually and can become worse over time. There may be periods of remission that can last for weeks or years.

- Researchers estimate that more than half a million people in the United States have Crohn's disease.

- Studies show that, over time, Crohn's disease has become more common in the United States and other parts of the world. Experts do not know the reason for this increase.

- Crohn's disease can develop in people of any age, though it's more likely to develop in people between the ages of twenty and twenty-nine.

- Those who have a family member with IBD, most often a sibling or parent, are at higher risk of developing an IBD themselves.

- Cigarette smokers are at high risk for Crohn's disease as well.

Possible complications from Crohn's Disease include the following:

Intestinal obstruction
- Crohn's disease can thicken the wall of the intestines.
- Over time, the thickened areas of the intestines can narrow, which can cause blockage.
- A partial or complete intestinal obstruction, also called a *bowel blockage*, can block the movement of food or stool through the intestines.

Fistulas
- Abnormal passages between two organs, or between an organ and the outside of the body.
- In Crohn's disease, inflammation can go through the wall of the intestines and create fistulas that may become infected.

Abscesses
- Painful, swollen, pus-filled pockets of infection.

Anal fissures
- Small tears in the anus that may cause itching, pain, or bleeding.

Ulcers
- Open sores in your mouth, intestines, anus, or perineum.

Malnutrition
- Develops when the body does not get the right amounts of vitamins, minerals, and nutrients it needs to maintain healthy tissues and organ function.

Additional inflammation
- Inflammation of the digestive tract may develop into inflammation of the joints, eyes, and skin as well.

Colon cancer
- If the Crohn's disease is in the large intestine, it may be more likely to develop into colon cancer.
- Ongoing treatment for Crohn's disease and remission may reduce the chances of it developing into colon cancer.
- Screening for colon cancer, which can include a colonoscopy with biopsies, may help to find cancer at an early stage in the absence of symptoms and improve the chance of curing the cancer.

3.2.6

Acid Reflux

- **Gastroesophageal Reflux (GER)**
- **Gastroesophageal Reflux Disease (GERD)**

Gastroesophageal Reflux (GER)
- Gastroesophageal reflux (GER) happens when your stomach contents come back up into your esophagus causing heartburn (also called acid reflux).

Gastroesophageal Reflux Disease (GERD)
- GERD is a more serious and long-lasting form of GER, specifically GER that occurs more than twice a week for a few weeks could be GERD.

- GERD can lead to more serious health problems over time. Medical attention is recommended.

- GERD affects about 20 percent of the US population.

- Anyone can develop GERD; some for unknown reasons. A person is more likely to develop GERD if he or she is:
    - Overweight or obese
    - Pregnant
    - Taking certain medicines
    - A smoker or regularly exposed to secondhand smoke

- <u>Without treatment, GERD can sometimes cause serious complications over time, such as:</u>

    Inflamed esophagus
    - Adults who have chronic esophagitis over many years are more likely to develop precancerous changes in the esophagus.

    Esophageal stricture
    - An esophageal stricture happens when your esophagus becomes too narrow. Esophageal strictures can lead to problems with swallowing.

    Respiratory problems
    - There is a risk of breathing stomach acid into the lungs, which can irritate the throat and lungs, causing respiratory problems.

    Barrett's esophagus
    - A small number of people with Barrett's esophagus develop a rare yet often deadly type of cancer of the esophagus.

CHAPTER 4

System Integration

4.1 Body Composition and Energy Systems ···················133
    4.1.1 What Body Weight Reveals and What It Doesn't ··········135
    4.1.2 Body Fat ··137
    4.1.3 Types of Fat Cells ···138
    4.1.4 What is the "Best" Way to Lose Body Fat? ················139
    4.1.5 How Many Calories Do I Need to Cut to Lose Weight? ·····141
    4.1.6 Eating Disorders ··143
    4.1.7 Calorie Burning Comparison for Exercise ················147
    4.1.8 Effect of Muscle Size on Lean Body Mass ················149
    4.1.9 Calories Burned by Adding Muscle ······················150
    4.1.10 Body Weight Stabilization ································152
    4.1.11 Body Function Stabilization ······························154
    4.1.12 Health Conditions Resulting from Chemical Imbalances ···156
    4.1.13 Metabolism ··158
    4.1.14 Basal Metabolic Rate (BMR) ······························159
    4.1.15 Energy Sources ···161
    4.1.16 Diabetes Mellitus and Hypoglycemia ······················165
    4.1.17 Aerobic and Anaerobic-Energy Systems ····················167
    4.1.18 Body Mass Index (BMI) ···································169
    4.1.19 BMI Formula ···170
    4.1.20 BMI Range Chart for Weight Categories ···················172
    4.1.21 Understanding Body Fat Percentage ······················173

4.2 Body Building · 175
- 4.2.1 How to Build Muscle Size and Strength · · · · · · · · · · · · · · · · · · · 177
- 4.2.2 Basic Muscle-Building Workout Charts · · · · · · · · · · · · · · · · · · · 179
- 4.2.3 Benefits of Warm-Ups and Cool-Downs · · · · · · · · · · · · · · · · · · 181
- 4.2.4 Are "Spot Reducing" Exercises Effective? · · · · · · · · · · · · · · · · · 183
- 4.2.5 Exercise Increases Abdominal Definition · · · · · · · · · · · · · · · · 184
- 4.2.6 Heat Conditions · 185
- 4.2.7 Wolff's Law · 188

4.3 Nutrition · 189
- 4.3.1 Calories and Kilocalories · 191
- 4.3.2 Caloric Values of the Three Main Nutrient Groups · · · · · · · · 192
- 4.3.3 Essential Nutrients · 193
- 4.3.4 Nutrient Density · 194
- 4.3.5 Six Nutrient Categories · 195
- 4.3.6 Symbols that Express the Quantities of Nutrients · · · · · · · · · · 196
- 4.3.7 Suggested Daily Intakes · 197
- 4.3.8 Water · 198
- 4.3.9 Carbohydrates · 199
- 4.3.10 Muscles & Protein · 203
- 4.3.11 Amino Acids · 205
- 4.3.12 Essential and Nonessential Amino Acids · · · · · · · · · · · · · · · · · · · 206
- 4.3.13 Fat and Fatty Acids · 207
- 4.3.14 Three Main Types of Fatty Acids · 209
- 4.3.15 Essential Fatty Acids · 211
- 4.3.16 "Bad" Fats · 213
- 4.3.17 Dietary Fat Intake · 215
- 4.3.18 Vitamins and Minerals · 217
- 4.3.19 Vitamin Descriptions · 220
- 4.3.20 Mineral Descriptions · 225
- 4.3.21 Free Radicals, Antioxidants, and CoQ10 · · · · · · · · · · · · · · · · · · · 228
- 4.3.22 Phytochemicals (Plant Chemicals) · 230

4.1
Body Composition and Energy Systems

4.1.1

What Body Weight Reveals and What It Doesn't

- **Body Weight**
- **Body Composition**
- **Contrasting Examples of Body Composition**

Body Weight
- Bathroom scales are very limited as to what they reveal.
- Knowing your body weight is important for health reasons, but for a more complete <u>understanding of your body</u>, you need more information about why your weight is what it shows on the scale.
- If you are trying to lose weight, it is not only how much weight you lose that matters but how much of the weight loss is fat loss.
- If you are into fitness, scales don't tell you what types of bodily tissues account for your body composition.

Body Composition
- Body composition analysis determines what percentage of your body weight is <u>lean body mass</u> and what percentage of your body weight is <u>body fat</u>.
- It can usually be determined by a certified personal fitness trainer or other medically qualified professional.
- Generally speaking, more lean body mass and less body fat is the goal, with occasional exceptions.
- Lean body mass and body fat percentages should correspond to a person's age and gender.
- A healthy percentage of lean body mass is a requirement for good fitness.

<u>Below are two contrasting examples of body composition and overall health for two males who weigh the same amount:</u>

Example 1:
- 68-year-old male
- 5 feet, 10 inches tall
- Gets <u>very little physical activity</u>

- Weighs 187 pounds, has a large waist, <u>and his percentage of body fat is very high</u>

- His 187-pound body weight is <u>unhealthy</u> for him.

Example 2:
- 68-year-old male
- 5 feet, 10 inches tall
- Leads a <u>very physical</u> lifestyle, is a weight lifter, does aerobics regularly

- Also weighs 187 pounds, is very lean and muscular, <u>and his percentage of body fat is very low</u>

- His 187-pound body weight is <u>healthy</u> for him

4.1.2

Body Fat

- **Adipose Tissue**
- **Subcutaneous Fat**
- **Visceral Fat**
- **Cellulite**

Adipose Tissue
- Loose connective tissue and the fatty tissue mass of the body.
- Primary function is to store energy in the form of fat.
- Also surrounds the internal organs to protect them and insulate the body.
- All the other tissues of the body are commonly referred to as lean body mass.

Subcutaneous Fat
- Adipose tissue that lies directly under the skin.
- It has nerves and blood vessels that bring oxygen to the skin.
- Acts as an energy source for the body.
- Protects the skin by acting as a cushion.

Visceral Fat
- Located deep within the body.
- Protects major organs such as the liver and heart by surrounding them to act as cushioning.
- Excess visceral fat is dangerous.

Cellulite
- Is **not** a special form of fat.
- It is simply a nonmedical name for subcutaneous fat and is usually more visible on women than on men.

4.1.3

Types of Fat Cells

- **White Fat Cells**
- **Brown Fat Cells**

White Fat Cells

- The most abundant type of fat cells, accounting for about 98–99 percent of the fat cells in the body.

- Stored throughout the body, this fat becomes most visible on our stomach, thighs, and hips.

Brown Fat Cells

- Considered to be the "good" fat, accounting for the remaining 1–2 percent of the fat cells in the body.

- When it comes to body weight, the really great thing about brown fat cells is that they are metabolically active, and instead of being stored as body fat, as is the case with white fat cells, they are actually burned for energy, and that generates body heat.

- Brown fat cells are packed with energy-producing mitochondria that also contain iron, which gives them their brown color.

- Infants are born with high amounts of brown fat cells (about 5 percent of their total body mass), and it is stored on the upper spine and shoulders to keep them warm. In adulthood, we lose some of these brown fat cells; however, we also store small amounts.

4.1.4

What is the "Best" Way to Lose Body Fat?

- **Caloric Intake**
- **Exercise**

Caloric Intake

- Your top priority must be to reduce your daily caloric intake. Only your physician can make the determination as to how many calories you can safely cut each day in a weight-loss program.

- It is also extremely important that you consume approximately eight glasses of water each day, as well as the recommended daily requirements from the three major food groups:

    1. Protein
    2. Carbohydrates
    3. Fats

Exercise

- Reducing your caloric intake is the single most important step for losing body fat, but aerobic exercise <u>must</u> be included in a healthy weight-loss program.

- Regardless of TV advertising or other types of marketing, the truth is that no special exercise or diet book can give you safer advice for weight loss than the recommendations above. Also, you cannot purchase a device that will shed pounds off your abs, or any other selected body part. Nature doesn't work that way.

- After checking with your doctor, use a certified personal fitness trainer to design a total fitness program that includes aerobics, a progressive weight-lifting program, proper dietary practices, and adequate rest.

4.1.5

How Many Calories Do I Need to Cut to Lose Weight?

To lose one to two pounds per week:
- You need to <u>reduce your intake of food</u> by about 500–1,000 calories daily.
- Generally, women will lose weight safely on an eating plan of about 1,000–1,200 calories daily.
- Generally, men will lose weight safely on an eating plan of about 1,200–1,600 calories daily.
- Your health, current weight, and exercise routines are among the other considerations for determining the amount of caloric intake that is safe for you. We strongly advise you to consult with your doctor before starting a weight-loss program.
- Never eat less than 800 calories per day unless you are under a doctor's supervision.

These are a few of the recommended ways to lose calories:
- <u>Eat smart</u>: Select foods that are lower in fat and added sugars.
- Exercise regularly.
- <u>Best:</u> Combine both of the above.
- Eat frequently: Four or five smaller meals per day (grazing) is ideal.
- Each meal should be 400–500 calories.
- Eating mini meals speeds up your metabolism, and your BMR.
- Breakfast really is the most important meal of the day, it gets your body off to a good start.
- If you just can't eat breakfast on a given day, eat fruit, or even a piece of bread.
- You will sabotage your body's ability to lose weight if you skip breakfast!

4.1.6

Eating Disorders

- Anorexia Nervosa
- Compulsive Exercising
- Fasting
- Starvation
- Ketosis
- Bulimia
- Yo-Yo Effect

- The only way to lose weight healthfully and successfully is to make proper changes to one's entire lifestyle.
- It is recommended that an individual seek medical attention when weight loss is a problem.
- In any effort to lose weight, be aware of and consult with a doctor to avoid the following eating disorders:

Anorexia Nervosa
- The most dangerous of all eating disorders.
- The victim suffers from an intense fear of gaining weight and resorts to various degrees of starvation.
- Characterized by a distorted body image whereby the person always feels fat, resulting in eating habits that lead to extreme weight loss.
- Eventually, if the victim is a woman, she will experience *amenorrhea* (the absence of monthly periods).

Compulsive Exercising
- An <u>extreme weight-loss disorder</u> that is particularly common among fashion models, dancers, gymnasts, and long-distance runners.
- In some cases, starvation leads to extreme undernourishment, where the victim's body weight may drop to seventy pounds or less.
- If left untreated, the victim may suffer from metabolic abnormalities, malnutrition, dehydration, electrolyte imbalance, seizures (convulsions), as well as many other physical problems and even death.
- This is a complex condition that is both psychological and physiological.

Fasting
- An unhealthy method to quickly lose weight.
- Involves a lack of food over a long period of time, although it may include the drinking of water only.
- Usually results in less fat being lost than would be the case on a low calorie diet due to the body's compromised rate of metabolism.
- Most of the weight that is lost during fasting is a result of water loss and lean body tissue (muscle, organ, and bone tissue).
- Usually the person who uses fasting as a method of losing weight eventually gains back all the weight that has been lost and frequently gains back even more weight.
- The progressive, negative effects of fasting result in a tremendous reduction in the body's energy output because the body strives to conserve its stores of fat and lean tissue.
- Seriousness increases as body organs begin to shrink, muscles begin to atrophy, and the body reduces its energy requirements.
- As the progression of harmful side effects continues, the body becomes extremely weak and tired as a result of the loss of minerals and water.
- To summarize, fasting is not only ineffective, but it is also dangerous.

Starvation
- <u>Differs from fasting because it is not a matter of choice</u>, whereas fasting is self-imposed. It is often a result of an <u>unwanted circumstance</u>, such as being denied of food.
- A serious condition where the victim suffers from a lack of food and water over a long period of time, resulting in unhealthy weight loss and dangerous changes in body chemistry (e.g., metabolism), as well as severe hunger.

Ketosis
- A dangerous build-up of ketones in the blood that offsets the body's normal acid–base balance.
- A serious condition usually resulting from fasting or starvation, a lack of food, and possibly water, over a long period of time as well as a diet that is <u>extremely low, or devoid of carbohydrates</u>.
- The body resorts to depleting its glycogen reserves for energy and then breaking down fat incompletely. It is this <u>incomplete breakdown of fat</u> that creates the build-up of ketones.
- The body reacts to this excessive ketone build-up by excreting the ketones into the urine, resulting in larger volumes of water being urinated and progressive dehydration in the person affected.
- The body resorts to not only breaking down fats for energy, but also protein tissue. This in turn causes additional complications to one's health and is a dangerous way to lose weight.

Bulimia
- An eating disorder that is characterized by a preoccupation with food, bulimia includes episodes of binge eating followed by fasting, self-induced vomiting (*emesis*), or the use of diuretics or laxatives and compulsive exercise.
- Bulimics may consume up to 5,000 calories in a one- to two-hour period.
- If left untreated, the victim may suffer from menstrual irregularities, potassium depletion, kidney failure, urinary tract infections, ulcers, and many other physical problems.
- Bulimics are usually easier to treat than anorexics because they are more likely to recognize that their behavior is abnormal and consequently are more likely to gain control over their abnormality.
- This eating disorder is usually worse when the bulimic eats alone; therefore, an excellent method of dealing with this problem is for the person to try to arrange to eat meals with other people. Alternatively, a family member or friend might arrange for the bulimic to eat with other people.

Yo-Yo Effect
- When weight loss is excessively fast and then that weight is regained after a period of time, often in greater amount than the weight that was lost.
- It becomes increasingly more difficult to lose weight after falling into a yo-yo effect pattern.

4.1.7

Calorie Burning Comparison for Exercise

- **<u>Aerobics</u>**
- **<u>Weight Lifting</u>**

Aerobics
- Aerobic exercises burn a far greater number of calories per minute during a workout than weight-lifting exercises.
- Aerobic exercises also <u>continue to burn calories briefly</u> following a workout.
- Aerobic exercises that are most effective include:
    - Treadmill
    - Elliptical
    - Bicycle
    - Stairs
    - Running
    - Walking
    - Swimming

Weight Lifting
- Where losing weight and keeping it off is the goal, a person should include a weight-lifting program to develop additional muscle tissue. (See Section 4.2.1
- The special benefit of muscle tissue is that it <u>continues to burn calories each and every second of the day, even while you sleep</u>.
- As you increase the percentage of muscle tissue in your body, you increase the rate at which your body burns calories.

Conclusion
- Aerobic exercise <u>burns calories faster</u>.
- Muscle tissue gained from weight lifting <u>burns calories continuously</u>.
- The best way to lose weight and to keep it off is to use a combination of weight lifting and aerobics, rather than using just one or the other.
- Finally, and very importantly, weight lifting adds the finishing touches by sculpting the body that you have worked so hard to slim down.

4.1.8

Effect of Muscle Size on Lean Body Mass

- **Lean Body Mass**
- **Body Composition**

Lean Body Mass
- Total body weight <u>minus</u> the weight of body fat determines a person's percentage of lean body mass.
- Essentially, <u>lean body mass</u> is composed of muscle, bone, glands, and all the other body tissues that are not fat.
- Your lean body mass is one component of your overall body composition.

Body composition
- The combination of two criteria:
    1. A person's percentage of <u>lean body mass</u>
    2. A person's percentage of <u>body fat</u>

Increasing muscle size increases lean body mass.
- See section 4.1.21 for <u>Understanding Body Fat Percentage</u>.

4.1.9

Calories Burned by Adding Muscle

- **Maintaining Muscle Tissue**
- **Myth Busting: Calories Burned by Adding Muscle**
- **Building Muscle Tissue**

Maintaining Muscle Tissue
- Muscle tissue requires high levels of energy in order to maintain and rebuild itself.
- An increase in muscle tissue can best be achieved by strength training.
- <u>Greater muscle size increases caloric consumption every second of every day</u>. Simply stated, the more muscle you have, the more calories you burn. This increase in caloric consumption is due to an increase in metabolism.
- Conversely, a decrease in muscle tissue results in a decrease in caloric consumption and metabolism.

Myth Busting: Calories Burned by Adding Muscle
- For many decades, there has been a popular <u>myth</u> that for every pound of muscle that you add, your body burns an extra <u>fifty to sixty</u> calories per day, even at rest. **This is a false concept**. In fact, muscle burns far less calories than had been previously believed.
- <u>Adding one pound of muscle results in burning about five to six extra calories per day, even at rest</u>. Therefore, you would need to add ten pounds of new muscle to burn about an extra fifty to sixty calories every day.
- In contrast, <u>one pound of fat</u> burns about <u>two to three calories per day</u>, even at rest.

Building Muscle Tissue
- With properly performed strength training programs, it is possible to add three to five pounds of muscle in three to four months, which translates to an extra caloric burn of approximately eighteen to thirty calories per day.
- If you are interested in building muscle (i.e., body building), see section 4.2.1

4.1.10

Body Weight Stabilization

- **Set-Point Theory**
- **Energy Balance Theory**
- **Food as Energy**
- **Thermal Effect of Food (TEF)**

Set-Point Theory
- States that everybody has an established normal body weight and that when the body deviates from that weight it tends to <u>adjust its metabolism to return to that weight</u>.

Energy Balance Theory
- The idea that <u>body weight will remain the same</u> providing that calorie intake equals calorie expenditure.
- The idea that positive calorie intake results in weight gain, and negative calorie intake results in weight loss.

Food as Energy
- Food is the body's fuel. It provides the potential to perform work and activities. As gasoline is the fuel that provides energy for a car, <u>food is the fuel that provides energy</u> for the body to perform all of its required functions.
- The energy from food is <u>measured by the calories</u> that are provided by the food's carbohydrates, proteins, and fats.

Thermal Effect of Food (TEF)
- Eating food requires the body to <u>expend energy</u> to digest, absorb, and metabolize that food.
- The amount of energy required for eating is thought to be about 10 percent of a person's daily food intake; therefore, if a person consumes two thousand calories a day, 10 percent (or two hundred calories) are required just to digest, absorb, and metabolize that food.

4.1.11

Body Function Stabilization

- **Homeostasis**
- **Blood Pressure**
- **Body Temperature**
- **Blood Sugar**

Homeostasis
- A normalization process that refers to the body's tendency to stabilize and balance its functions.
- This continuous process works to keep the body's internal environment operating normally in spite of constant external changes.
- The stabilization process is the primary function of most organs.
- Examples of the homeostatic function of organs include:
    - Regulation of blood pressure
    - Regulation of body temperature
    - Regulation of blood sugar levels
- These conditions are regulated by negative feedback. When blood pressure, body temperature, or blood sugar vary from normal levels, the body automatically works to counteract the abnormality and reestablish normal levels.

Blood Pressure
- Within the circulatory system, *baroreceptors* (pressure sensors), help to keep blood pressure at nearly constant levels by sending rapid negative feedback to the brain that results in causing the heart rate to decrease and blood pressure to decrease.
- The body contains two other, slower acting systems to regulate blood pressure:
    1. The heart releases *atrial natriuretic peptide* (a substance secreted by heart muscle cells) when blood pressure is too high.
    2. The kidneys sense and correct low blood pressure with the *renin-angiotensin system* (a hormone system that is involved in the regulation of the plasma sodium concentration and arterial blood pressure).

Body Temperature (Too Hot or Too Cold)
- As discussed above, homeostasis is the process that normalizes body temperature, whether the body is too hot, or too cold.
- Homeostasis is regulated by the *hypothalamus*, a part of the brain.
- It should be noted that the hypothalamus is also responsible for other metabolic processes and activities of the autonomic nervous system that do not relate to body temperature, and therefore not discussed.
- One of the most important functions of the hypothalamus is to link the nervous system to the endocrine system via the pituitary gland, which in turn releases hormones to stimulate or inhibit the secretion of pituitary hormones to regulate body temperature.

Blood Sugar
- When a body's blood sugar levels are too high, it counteracts by causing the pancreas (which is part of the endocrine system) to produce *insulin* to enable the blood sugar level to return back to normal.

- When a body's blood sugar levels are too low, it counteracts by causing the pancreas to produce *glucagon* to enable the blood sugar level to return back to normal.

4.1.12

Health Conditions Resulting from Chemical Imbalances

- Hypokalemia
- Hyperkalemia
- Hyperthyroidism
- Hypothyroidism

Hypokalemia
- Low blood-potassium level
- Symptoms include, but are not limited to, muscular weakness, cardiac arrhythmias, shallow breathing, and paralysis.
- Can be caused by kidney failure, diarrhea, and vomiting as well as disease such as Cushing's syndrome.

Hyperkalemia
- High blood-potassium level
- Symptoms include, but are not limited to, cardiac arrhythmias, cardiac arrest, paralysis, and muscular weakness.
- It can also be caused by kidney disease or Addison's disease.

Hyperthyroidism
- Also called overactive thyroid, is when the thyroid gland makes more thyroid hormones than your body needs.
- The thyroid is a small, butterfly-shaped gland in the front of your neck.
- Thyroid hormones control the way the body uses energy, so they affect nearly every organ in your body, even the way your heart beats.
- If left untreated, hyperthyroidism can cause serious problems with the heart, bones, muscles, menstrual cycle, and fertility.

Hypothyroidism
- Also called underactive thyroid, is when the thyroid gland doesn't make enough thyroid hormones to meet your body's needs.
- Without enough thyroid hormones, many of your body's functions slow down.

4.1.13

Metabolism

- Metabolism is a combination of physiological and chemical processes that are required by the body in order to supply the energy that is necessary to maintain life.

- As we age there is a natural and continuous decline in our metabolism, along with other degenerative processes.

- To counter the decline in metabolism, we need to <u>increase the percentage of muscle tissue in our bodies</u>.

- The best way to add muscle tissue is to lift weights.
    - <u>See Section 4.2.1 How to Build Muscle Size and Strength</u>

    - **To avoid confusion**, aerobic exercises such as:
      running, walking, treadmill, stepper, elliptical, swimming, and bicycle <u>do not</u> add substantial amounts of muscle tissue.
    - However, these exercises do offer a wide variety of cardiorespiratory and disease prevention benefits.

4.1.14

Basal Metabolic Rate (BMR)

- BMR is the <u>energy requirement of your body at rest</u> that is necessary to maintain normal body functions such as heartbeat, respiration, and body temperature.

- An individual's BMR uses approximately 60–70 percent of the body's energy requirement. For example, if a person requires 2,000 calories per day, approximately 1,200–1,400 will be needed to support the BMR.

- BMR reaches its highest level for both males and females at age twenty. Then it decreases by 2 percent each decade for the rest of one's life. At age thirty, the BMR operates at 98 percent efficiency; at age forty it operates at 96 percent efficiency. At age seventy, it operates at 90 percent efficiency. This decline continues throughout life.

- Besides age, factors that affect BMR include: gender, height, diet, exercise, environmental conditions, and much more.

- <u>The amount of muscle mass that we have helps to determine our basal metabolic rate (BMR).</u> After we reach the age of twenty, we lose about one-half pound of muscle mass per year, our BMR decreases, and we burn fewer and fewer calories each day. That results in a tendency to put on weight. A decrease in physical activity is the primary cause for this muscle loss.

- The good news is that we can add muscle mass as we get older, and that will increase our BMR, which will increase the number of calories that we burn while at rest. Burning more calories while resting makes it easier to lose weight and to maintain a healthy body weight.

- The very best way to slow down the decline in BMR is to add muscle mass. Start a weight-lifting program designed for you by a certified personal fitness trainer.

- Simply stated, more muscle tissue translates to more calories burned at rest every day. A major benefit of the faster metabolism is the increased ability to lose weight or maintain a healthy weight.

4.1.15

Energy Sources

- Substrate
- Phosphagens (ATP & CP)
    - Synthesis
    - Hydrolysis
- Enzymes
- Endorphins
- Adrenaline (Epinephrine)
- Insulin
- Lactate (Lactic Acid)
    - Pyruvate

Substrate
- A fuel source for energy metabolism that is made up of carbohydrates (glucose) and fat (fatty acids).
- This fuel source is used by the cells of the body to produce most of the ATP supply.
    - See the other Energy Sources on the following pages.

Phosphagens
- The body's two high-energy storage compounds, *adenosine triphosphate* (ATP) and *creatine phosphate* (CP), are high-energy phosphate molecules that can be immediately metabolized to increase cell function.
- These phosphate molecules are mostly stored in muscle tissue.
- For a highly trained athlete who is doing high-intensity activity, the combined phosphagen stores of ATP and CP have only enough energy to last about ten seconds.
- For a nonathletic person doing high-intensity activity, the available energy would be somewhat less than ten seconds.

Adenosine Triphosphate (ATP)
- This high-energy phosphate molecule is required in order to provide energy for cells to function.
- The body produces ATP both aerobically (with oxygen) and anaerobically (without oxygen).
- Much more ATP is produced during aerobic activity than during anaerobic activity.
- To further understand the dynamics of ATP, one must understand the terms <u>synthesis</u> and <u>hydrolysis</u>:

    - **Synthesis** is when two or more chemical compounds, or chemical elements, combine to form a more complex compound. ATP transports chemical energy within cells and is vital to the synthesis of nucleic acids. <u>The human body stores about 0.1 mole of ATP</u>.
    - **Hydrolysis** refers to a chemical reaction that must include water, wherein one chemical compound produces another compound. The hydrolysis of two hundred to three hundred moles of ATP daily are required to supply energy to the body's cells. Therefore, 0.1 mole of ATP must be recycled two to three thousand times daily.
- Because large quantities of ATP cannot be stored, the consumption of ATP must be directly related to its synthesis.

Creatine Phosphate (CP)
- This high-energy phosphate molecule that is stored in the cells is used instantly to resynthesize ATP.

Enzymes
- Organic compounds that are composed mostly of proteins, <u>enzymes are used in the process of digestion</u>.
- They act as catalysts to bring about a series of chemical breakdowns of complex compounds into simpler substances.
- The end result is the production of energy for the body's needs.

Endorphins
- A natural substance produced by the cells of the body that have morphine-like characteristics, endorphins relieve pain, improve mood, and are also involved in other bodily functions.
- Many people who have been exercising heavily over an extended period of time, such as body builders and long-distance runners, enjoy the benefits of increased levels of endorphins. They experience an elevated feeling of energy, tranquility, strength, and well-being.

Adrenaline (Epinephrine)
- A hormone produced by the adrenal glands that is secreted directly into the bloodstream, adrenaline results in a noticeable increase in energy.
- <u>Some of its most important functions include the following</u>:
    - Increasing the speed and force of each heartbeat, which enables the heart to work harder.
    - Dilating (opening) airways to allow more air to pass through, which improves breathing, and therefore, enables the body to work harder.
    - Enabling more blood to reach the muscles, which increases their ability to work harder.

Insulin
- In the pancreas there is a small group of cells called the *Islets of Langerhans* (also called the *Islands of Langerhans*), and they produce the hormone insulin.
- Insulin is necessary to control the proper levels of glucose (blood sugar) within the cells of the body.
- Insulin enables other cells to convert glucose into energy.
- Insulin must be available in just the right amounts, neither too much nor too little, to keep glucose at the proper levels.
- The energy derived from glucose is available to use immediately or at a later time.
- A deficiency in the production or use of insulin causes an elevation in the levels of glucose (blood sugar) and may result in the medical condition known as diabetes.
- Conversely, an excess of insulin within the cells of the body causes a decrease in the levels of glucose (blood sugar) and may result in the condition known as hypoglycemia.
- A further understanding of insulin, diabetes, and hypoglycemia is found in section 4.1.16.

Lactate (Lactic Acid)
- A multifunctional chemical that has three major purposes, lactate responds to aerobic and anaerobic exercises by fueling the muscles, delaying fatigue, and preventing injury.
- The body does not store *lactic acid*. Instead, it produces lactate, which is lactic acid minus one proton.
- When the body doesn't have enough oxygen to continue an exercise, it converts *pyruvate* (an intermediate compound in the metabolism of carbohydrates, proteins, and fats.) into lactate to fuel its muscles. If the muscles did not produce sufficient amounts of lactate while doing high-intensity exercise, the muscles would fatigue more quickly.

4.1.16

Diabetes Mellitus and Hypoglycemia

- **Diabetes Mellitus**
- **Type 1 and Type 2 Diabetes**
- **Diabetes and Exercise**
- **Hypoglycemia**

Diabetes Mellitus
- <u>The inability of the pancreas to provide sufficient production and utilization of the hormone insulin.</u>
- Insulin enables glucose to be transferred from the blood and to enter into the body's cells, a process that helps to maintain normal blood glucose levels. In the nondiabetic individual, eating determines the amount of insulin secreted by the pancreas in order to maintain normal blood sugar levels.
- Diabetes is a chronic metabolic disorder for which there is no cure.
- Diabetes is a disease, however, that can be controlled.
- If left untreated, it may result in circulatory problems, kidney disease, blindness, or death.
- The two types of diabetes mellitus are Type 1 and Type 2.

Type 1 Diabetes
- Type 1 diabetics are either born with it or develop it in their childhood.
- For the Type 1 diabetic, the <u>pancreas produces little or no insulin</u>. This individual is <u>insulin dependent</u> and must take insulin injections on a daily basis.
- For the 5 percent of diabetics who are Type 1 diabetics, this is a lifelong condition.

Type 2 Diabetes
- About 95 percent of all diabetics are Type 2 diabetics.
- Type 2 diabetics usually develop the disease in adulthood.
- For the Type 2 diabetic, the body produces an insufficient supply of insulin, but the individual can control blood glucose (sugar) levels through diet, exercise, and oral medications.
- In Type 2 Diabetes, the individual is <u>not insulin dependent</u>.

Diabetes and Exercise
- Exercise can lower a diabetic's glucose levels.
- Exercise increases the entry of glucose into the cells; however, if the diabetic exercises too much, eats too little, or takes too much insulin, it can create an abnormally low blood sugar level. This condition may cause the diabetic to experience an episode of hypoglycemia.

Hypoglycemia
- Hypoglycemia is a glucose deficiency in the blood.
- Most cases of hypoglycemia affect people with insulin-dependent diabetes mellitus.
- It is generally caused by too much insulin, too little glucose, or too much exercise.
- The typical symptoms of hypoglycemia are feeling faint, loss of consciousness, excessive fatigue, seizures, lightheadedness, shakiness, sweating, headache, irritability, slurred speech, poor circulation, or butterflies in the stomach.
- Hypoglycemia is a serious condition because the brain needs glucose for proper functioning and lengthy periods of insufficient glucose may permanently impair the health of the brain.

4.1.17

Aerobic and Anaerobic-Energy Systems

- **Aerobic Exercises**
- **Anaerobic Exercises**
- **Anaerobic Threshold**

- Energy used for muscle contraction is derived from three primary energy systems.
- These systems are all responsible for producing adenosine triphosphate (ATP), the body's primary energy source.
- ATP is responsible for the contraction and force that a muscle produces.

Aerobic Exercises
- The term *aerobic* means with oxygen.
- An exercise is aerobic when sufficient amounts of oxygen are available to the body's cells to enable fatty acids, glucose, and glycogen to produce ATP.

Anaerobic Exercises
- The term *anaerobic* means without oxygen.
- An exercise is anaerobic when insufficient amounts of oxygen are available to the body's cells to enable the body to produce ATP.
- The body relies upon the two anaerobic-energy systems for the production of ATP:
    1. Phosphagens to produce ATP.
    2. Glucose and glycogen to produce ATP.

Anaerobic Threshold
- The point during high-intensity activity at which the cardiovascular system can no longer meet the body's demand for oxygen by utilizing the aerobic energy system
- Consequently, this lack of oxygen causes the body to rely primarily on its anaerobic-energy systems.

4.1.18

Body Mass Index (BMI)

- BMI is an <u>estimate</u> of body fat and is a good gauge of the risks for diseases that can be related to an excess of body fat.
- The higher a person's BMI, the higher the risk for certain diseases such as heart disease, high blood pressure, Type 2 diabetes, gallstones, breathing problems, certain cancers, and many other diseases.
- Although BMI can be used for most men and women, it does have some limits.
- BMI may overestimate body fat in athletes and others who have a muscular build.
- BMI may underestimate body fat in older persons and others who have lost muscle.

4.1.19

BMI Formula

Weight in Kilograms ÷ Height in Meters^2

Example using:
- A weight of 175 pounds,
- A height of 5'5" (65 inches)

Step 1: Convert Pounds to Kilograms
- Weight in pounds ÷ 2.2
- 175 pounds ÷ 2.2 = 79.54 kilograms

Step 2: Convert Inches to Meters:
- Height in inches x 0.0254
- 65 inches x 0.0254 = 1.65 meters

Step 3: Convert Meters to Meters^2
- 1.65 x 1.65 = 2.72 meters^2

Step 4: Calculate BMI
- Weight in kilograms ÷ height in meters^2
- 79.54 kilograms ÷ 2.72 meters^2 = 29.24

This calculation determined that the example person's **BMI is 29.24**, and therefore **overweight**.

See the chart in section 4.1.20 for healthy BMI ranges.

4.1.20

BMI Range Chart for Weight Categories

Weight Category	BMI Range	Percent Above & Below Normal Weight
Normal Weight	18.5 to 24.9	0%
Overweight	25 to 29.9	10 to 19.9%
Obese	30 to 39.9	20 to 40%
Extremely Obese	> 40	> 40%
Underweight	< 18.5	10% or more under normal body weight

- **Overfat** is a better term than <u>overweight or obese</u> because it refers to the amount of fat in one's body that is above normal levels. The fat percentage reflects a more accurate assessment of one's general health than weight does.

4.1.21

Understanding Body Fat Percentage

Very Lean Percent of Body Fat for Women
- Less than 17%

Very Lean Percent of Body Fat for Men
- Less than 8%

Healthy Percent of Body Fat for Women
- From 18 to 22%

Healthy Percent of Body Fat for Men
- From 8 to 12%

Obese Percent of Body Fat for Women
- From 30% or more

Obese Percent of Body Fat for Men
- From 20% or more

Ideal Percent of Body Fat for Women
- From 17 to 27%

Ideal Percent of Body Fat for Men
- From 10 to 16%

4.2 Body Building

4.2.1

How to Build Muscle Size and Strength

Theory
- Muscles grow in size and strength when they are stimulated by exercises that use proper progressive <u>increases in weight</u>, as well as proper <u>increases in repetitions</u>, and are continued over a prolonged period of time, as in months or years.
- The most effective way to accomplish these muscle gains is to lift free weights or use weight-lifting machines.

Technique
- The following example explains the basic technique for increasing muscle size and strength. Be sure to get clearance from your physician if you have any condition that might put you at risk. Also, if you are over fifty years of age, you should consult a physician for clearance.

    1. The exerciser wants to increase muscle strength and size in her legs.
    2. The exercise that stimulates the greatest amount of muscle tissue throughout the legs is the squat (or leg press on a machine).
    3. If you are a beginner, you need to select a weight that allows you to comfortably perform eight to twelve repetitions, using proper form, for three sets.
    4. If you can do more than twelve repetitions, then the weight is too light.
    5. If you can't do eight repetitions, then the weight is too heavy.
    6. If you can do between eight and twelve repetitions, then the weight is correct.
    7. After you've performed the first set, wait sixty seconds, and repeat two more times for a total of three sets. Use the same technique for your next exercise.
    8. About every two weeks, try to increase the weight and repetitions (by no more than 5 percent). Wait longer if you struggle to make these increases.

4.2.2

Basic Muscle-Building Workout Charts

- Legs
- Buttocks
- Back
- Chest
- Arms
- Abdominals

Exercise Machines	For These Muscles	Repetitions	Sets	Times Per Week
Leg Press	Legs (Quadriceps) & Buttocks (Glutei)	8–12	1–3	2–3
Leg Extension	Legs (Quadriceps)	8–12	1–3	2–3
Leg Curl	Legs (Hamstrings)	8–12	1–3	2–3
Pulldown & Rowing	Back (Latissimus dorsi)	8–12	1–3	2–3
Bench Press & Pec-Deck	Chest (Pectoralis major)	8–12	1–3	2–3
Triceps Press	Arms (Triceps)	8–12	1–3	2–3
Biceps Curl	Arms (Biceps)	8–12	1–3	2–3
Abdominal	Abdominals (Rectus abdominis) & (External oblique) & (Internal oblique) & (Transverse abdominis)	8–12	1–3	2–3

4.2.3

Benefits of Warm-Ups and Cool-Downs

- A necessary part of a workout routine, warming up and cooling down muscles increase safety and performance. Please be sure to follow these practices.

Warm-Up
- Gradually increases metabolic activity such as oxygen consumption, which in turn increases cardiorespiratory performance.
- Gradually increases body temperature, which increases muscle performance and reduces the risk of injury.
- Gradually increases nerve response for motor unit activity.
- Gradually increases blood flow, which reduces the risk of a heart trauma.
- Gradually increases a positive psychological response, which enables an easier progression to more intensive exercise.

Cool-Down
- To reduce bodily risk after your work out, it is essential that you cool down your body for at least five to ten minutes by <u>performing low level aerobic exercise</u>.
- You can use any aerobic exercise machine, but gradually taper the intensity so that when you finish, your aerobic effort is equivalent to a very slow walk.

Benefits:
- Reduces the possibility of blood pooling, a sudden drop in blood pressure, lightheadedness, dizziness, and fainting.
- Reduces the possibility of muscle spasms and cramping.
- Reduces the amounts of beneficial hormones such as endorphins that are produced from vigorous exercise.
- It is very important to lower the amounts of these hormones to reduce the risk of cardiac rhythm irregularities.

4.2.4

Are "Spot Reducing" Exercises Effective?

Spot Reducing

- <u>Targeting a specific body part in order to lose weight in that area.</u>

- A technique often used during weight training in an effort to make the abdominals, thighs, butt, or triceps smaller.

<u>Why Spot Reducing Does Not Work</u>

- All exercises, <u>especially aerobic exercises</u>, play a role in the reduction of body fat.

- Where body fat is lost is determined by your genetics—not by the choice of exercise, the weight used, the number of repetitions, or the number of times a week that you exercise.

- You cannot use abdominal exercises only to reduce your waist size, for example. Even by doing hundreds of sit-ups every day, or by using abdominal exercise devices, you will not shrink your waist size.

- When you perform a weight-training exercise on a body part, you actually increase its muscle size; you do not lose size.

4.2.5

Exercise Increases Abdominal Definition

If you are interested in <u>defining your abdominals</u>, or as many people express it, "<u>building your six-pack</u>," <u>then follow the two steps below to achieve the best possible results:</u>

1. Reduce waist size using a combination of aerobic exercise and disciplined dietary habits. Muscle definition will never be visible if your abs are covered with fat.

2. Use resistance exercise such as weight lifting to build abdominal muscle.

Remember: Weight lifting exercises alone will not reduce belly fat nor give you abdominal muscle definition. You must remove belly fat to make your developed abs visible.

4.2.6

Heat Conditions

- **Dehydration**
- **Heat Cramps**
- **Heat Exhaustion**
- **Heat Stroke**
- **Hypochloremia**
- **Hyponatremia**
- **Hypernatremia**

Common sense exercise techniques include:

- Maintaining adequate hydration, perhaps the most important preventative measure that you can implement.
- Understanding your body and not trying to push beyond your capabilities.
- Adjusting your exercise plan to consider weather conditions.
- Consuming proper nutrition at the appropriate time prior to your specific exercise.

These suggestions are **not** to be construed as our personal prescription for your particular needs, but rather a general outline of some of the usual recommendations by most sports health specialists.

The potential health consequences resulting from exercise include a variety of heat conditions outlined below (though it should be noted that these conditions can also be caused by reasons other than exercise).

Dehydration
- The excessive loss of water as a result of perspiration.
- In preparation for exercising or an athletic competition, an individual should adhere to proper fluid replacement guidelines for exercise and be sure to consume adequate amounts of water before, during, and after the activity.

Heat Cramps
- Painful muscle spasms that occur during or after strenuous physical activity, heat cramps are considered a mild, heat-related illness.

Heat Exhaustion
- This is the most common heat-related illness and usually results from excessive exercise in hot, humid weather.
- Symptoms include profuse sweating with fluid and electrolyte loss, drop in blood pressure, lightheadedness, nausea, vomiting, decreased coordination, and fainting (*syncope*).

Heat Stroke
- This is the most serious heat-related illness and is caused by a heat overload, or the inability of the body to dissipate heat.
- Symptoms include body temperatures in excess of 105 degrees Fahrenheit, dry red skin, changing levels of consciousness, comas, seizures, and in extreme cases, death.

Hypochloremia
- Low blood-chloride level
- The symptoms include, but are not limited to, breathing difficulty, alkalosis, and muscle spasms.
- It can be caused by dehydration, diarrhea, and vomiting.

Hyponatremia
- Low blood-sodium level
- The symptoms include, but are not limited to, headache, confusion, muscular weakness, and hypotension.
- It can be caused by sweating, drinking abnormally huge amounts of water, use of some diuretics, and diarrhea as well as disease, such as Addison's disease.

Hypernatremia
- High blood-sodium level
- The symptoms include, but are not limited to, coma, confusion, and nervous system abnormalities.
- It can be caused by not drinking enough water, by diseases like *diabetes insipidus* or Cushing's syndrome, or by the use of salt tablets, usually taken before athletic events.
- Salt tablets can cause or worsen a dehydration problem by causing water to be drawn out of the body tissues, where it is most needed, and into the stomach, which eventually leads to its elimination.
- Salt is an essential mineral and most diets contain more than a sufficient amount. Therefore, no supplementation is necessary for normal, healthy people.

4.2.7

Wolff's Law

- Wolff's Law states that bones strengthen in direct response to the proportion of work or exercise that they are subjected to over a continuous period of time. Conversely, bones will weaken in the absence of work or exercise.

- Resistance exercises such as weight lifting increase muscle tissue size while simultaneously forcing the bones to become denser and stronger to compensate for the additional muscle tissue gain.

- Physicians often recommend progressive weight training to address the problem of osteoporosis.

4.3 Nutrition

4.3.1

Calories and Kilocalories

Calorie
- The amount of heat energy required to raise the temperature of <u>one gram</u> of water by one degree centigrade, also referred to as a *small calorie*.

Kilocalorie
- The amount of heat energy required to raise the temperature of <u>one kilogram</u> of water by one degree centigrade.
- Also referred to as a *large calorie* or the word <u>*Calorie* spelled with a capital "C."</u>
- One kilocalorie is equivalent to one thousand small calories.

4.3.2

Caloric Values of the Three Main Nutrient Groups

- Carbohydrates — 1 gram = 4 calories
- Proteins — 1 gram = 4 calories
- Fats — 1 gram = 9 calories

4.3.3

Essential Nutrients

Certain nutrients that are vital to bodily functions cannot be produced by the body and can only be obtained from food. Four examples are:

1. Essential Amino Acids (see section 4.3.12)
2. Essential Fatty Acids (see section 4.3.15)
3. Essential Vitamins (see section 4.3.18)
4. Essential Minerals (see section 4.3.18)

4.3.4

Nutrient Density

- A measure of the amount of nutrients versus the number of calories for a particular food is called *nutrient density*.
- <u>Foods that are nutrient-dense provide more nutrients than calories.</u>
- Foods that contain more calories than nutrients are labeled as *empty calories*.

4.3.5

Six Nutrient Categories

1. Carbohydrates
2. Proteins (Amino Acids)
3. Fats
4. Water
5. Vitamins
6. Minerals

4.3.6

Symbols that Express the Quantities of Nutrients

IU (International Units)

g (Grams)

mg (Milligrams)

mcg (µg) (Micrograms)

AI (Adequate Intake)

4.3.7

Suggested Daily Intakes

- **Carbohydrates**
- **Proteins**
- **Fats**

Carbohydrates
- Consume 55–60 percent of your daily calories from carbohydrates.
- For the average diet, this amounts to approximately 350–400 grams.
- No less than 125 grams of carbohydrates should be consumed each day.

Proteins
- Consume 12–20 percent of your daily calories from proteins.
- For the average diet, this amounts to approximately fifty to seventy grams.
- Consuming extra protein does not help to build muscle faster. In fact, consuming extra protein can result in the addition of extra body fat and cause damage to certain organs of the body.

Fats
- Consume 25–30 percent of your daily calories from fat.
- For the average diet, this amounts to approximately thirty to sixty-five grams.
- No more than ten grams of this fat should be <u>saturated</u>.

4.3.8

Water

- **Water Requirements**
- **Water Functions**

Water Requirements
- Recommended intake of water is eight glasses per day (eight ounces per glass) for people who are sedentary.
- Those who engage in vigorous activities, whether for work, pleasure, or exercise, must increase their intake accordingly.

Water Functions
- The body is composed of about 60 percent water. It is essential for life.
- Without water the body would survive for only a few days. It is necessary for chemical reactions in the body.
- Water is a component of body fluids that are used to transport required chemicals throughout the body and to remove by-products from the body.
- Water helps to lubricate joints, and it also protects tissues and organs of the body from shock.
- Water also helps to maintain proper body temperature.

4.3.9

Carbohydrates

- **Simple Carbohydrates**
- **Complex Carbohydrates**
- **Food Examples**
- **Glucose**
- **Glycogen**
- **Glycemic Index**

- Carbohydrates are vital nutrients that supply the body with energy.
- Chemically, a carbohydrate is a compound of carbon, hydrogen, and oxygen (CHO), containing twice as much hydrogen as oxygen.
- Carbohydrates are one of the three main constituents of food (the others are proteins and fats).
- One gram of carbohydrates equals four calories.

Simple Carbohydrates

a) Monosaccharides:
- Glucose (simple sugar)
- Fructose (fruit sugar)
- Galactose (milk sugar)

b) Disaccharides:
- Sucrose (table sugar)
- Lactose (milk sugar)
- Maltose (malt sugar)

Complex carbohydrates

   a)   Polysaccharides (starch, glycogen)

See food examples of simple and complex carbohydrates on the next page.

Food Examples

Simple carbohydrates:
- Corn sweetener
- Syrup
- Malt syrup
- Corn syrup
- High-fructose corn syrup
- Dextrose
- Maltose
- Sucrose
- Fructose
- Glucose
- Lactose
- Molasses
- Honey
- White Sugar
- Brown sugar
- Soda
- White bread
- Cookies
- Donuts
- Candy Bars
- Fudge
- Flavored Water
- Ice cream

Complex carbohydrates (or starches):
- Seeds
- Nuts
- Legumes
- Whole-Grain Breads
- Whole-Grain Pastas
- Brown rice
- Corn
- Wheat
- Barley
- Fruits and Vegetables
- Oats
- Quinoa
- Dairy
- Low-fat yogurt
- Skim milk

Glucose
- **All** carbohydrates, both *simple* and *complex*, are converted to *glucose* (blood sugar).
- Glucose is a ***simple sugar*** and the main source of energy to supply the cells of the body and the brain.
- The digestion of *complex carbohydrates* releases glucose into your bloodstream slower and more evenly than when digesting *simple carbohydrates*.

Glycogen
- Unused glucose is stored in the liver and muscles as *glycogen*, and glycogen can be quickly converted back to glucose to meet the body's energy needs.

Glycemic Index
- Used to classify approximately six hundred foods on the basis of how fast a carbohydrate food is digested into glucose, and how that digestive process causes the blood sugar to elevate.

4.3.10

Muscles & Protein

- Protein Composition
- General Protein Requirements
- Protein Requirements for Athletes
- Protein Supplements
- Protein Cautions

Protein Composition
- The body's muscle tissue is comprised of approximately 20–25 percent protein and 75–80 percent water.

General Protein Requirements
- In modern countries, the average diet supplies more protein than is required for maintaining and increasing muscle growth.
- The average adult requires <u>per day</u> about <u>one gram of protein for every 2.2 pounds of bodyweight</u>. <u>For example, a 175-pound adult needs eighty grams of protein per day</u> (175 pounds ÷ 2.2 grams/pound = 80 grams), which is less than three ounces of protein a day.
- After the growth years, adults lose about a half-pound of muscle a year, regardless of their protein consumption, unless they perform an adequate amount of progressive resistance exercise. Just consuming extra protein does not increase muscle size.
- Only progressive resistance exercise can increase muscle strength and size, and that's providing that a balanced diet is followed and sleep requirements are met. Additionally, a person's genetics play an important role in muscle development.

Protein Requirements for Athletes
- As it relates to athletes, the body's protein requirement does vary based on the level of prolonged physical exertion.
- Typically, the daily protein requirements for <u>athletes</u> are between <u>1.2 and 1.7 grams of protein</u> for every 2.2 pounds of bodyweight, which is higher than for the average adult.
- <u>Calculating the daily protein requirements for a 175-pound adult athlete requires additional steps after finding the daily grams for the average adult:</u>
    1) 175 pounds ÷ 2.2 = 80 grams (which is the required number of grams of protein daily for the average adult).
    2) Using the accepted ranges for athletes, which are 1.2 to 1.7 grams of protein a day, see (a) & (b) below:
        a) <u>80 x 1.2</u> = 96 grams, which is 3.4 ounces of protein required at the <u>lower level</u>.
        b) <u>80 x 1.7</u> = 136 grams, which is 4.8 ounces of protein required at the <u>higher level</u>.

Protein Supplements
- The use of protein supplements is a common practice, especially among weight lifters, runners, and people in certain other sports where there is a high priority on muscle strength, size, endurance, and appearance.
- As previously stated, in modern countries, the average diet supplies more protein than is required for maintaining and increasing muscle growth.

Protein Cautions
- Whenever a person consumes more protein than the body can use:
    - The extra amino acids are stored in the body as fat.
    - The extra protein places a strain on the kidneys.

4.3.11

Amino Acids

- **Essential**
- **Nonessential**

- Amino acids are considered to be the building blocks of protein.

- There are <u>twenty amino acids</u> that combine to form this vital nutrient that is responsible for the building and repairing of body tissue.

- Each of the twenty amino acids fall into one of two categories:

    - **Essential amino acids:** cannot be made by the body and must be obtained from diet.

    - **Nonessential amino acids:** can be made by the body.

See section 4.3.12 for a list of the essential amino acids and the nonessential amino acids.

4.3.12

Essential and Nonessential Amino Acids

Essential Amino Acids	Nonessential Amino Acids
1. Histidine (his)	1. Alanine (ala)
2. Isoleucine (ile)	2. Arginine (arg)
3. Leucine (leu)	3. Asparagine (asn)
4. Lysine (lys)	4. Aspartic Acid (asp)
5. Methionine (met)	5. Cysteine (cys)
6. Phenylalanine (phe)	6. Glutamic Acid (glu)
7. Threonine (thr)	7. Glutamine (gln)
8. Tryptophan (trp)	8. Glycine (gly)
9. Valine (val)	9. Proline (pro)
	10. Serine (ser)
	11. Tyrosine (tyr)

4.3.13

Fat and Fatty Acids

- **Fat**
- **Fatty Acids**
- **Lipids**

Fat
- Fat is a vital nutrient that is necessary for proper functioning of the body and energy storage. It supplies the body with energy for daily activities as well as for exercises that are low in intensity and long in duration (e.g., aerobics).
- Fat also carries the four fat-soluble vitamins (A, D, E, and K), insulates the body, and cushions to protect internal organs.
- Fat is one of the three main constituents of food (the other two are protein and carbohydrates).
- Fat is also needed to supply essential fatty acids, which are necessary for growth and protection against diseases.

Fatty Acids
- Fatty acids are the building blocks of fat.
- Chemically, fat is a compound that consists mostly of carbon and hydrogen.
- Essential fatty acids are not produced by the body and must be obtained from diet.

Lipids
- A group of fatty substances that include cholesterol and triglycerides, lipids are vital nutrients that are a necessary part of every cell.
- Lipids store energy, supply energy to the body when needed, protect internal organs, and carry the four fat-soluble vitamins (A, D, E, and K).
- Lipids are also characterized by the fact that they are insoluble in water.

4.3.14

Three Main Types of Fatty Acids

- **Saturated Fatty Acid**
- **Monounsaturated Fatty Acid**
- **Polyunsaturated Fatty Acid**

Saturated Fatty Acids
- A fatty acid that carries the <u>maximum number of hydrogen atoms</u> and is therefore *saturated*.
- Saturated fats increase LDL cholesterol levels and promote artery-clogging fatty deposits.
- Saturated fatty acids are solid at room temperature and mainly come from animal foods and can also be made from vegetable oils through a process called *hydrogenation*.
- <u>Some common saturated fats are</u>:
    - butter
    - milk fat
    - beef fat (tallow, suet)
    - chicken fat
    - cream
    - pork fat (lard)
    - stick margarine
    - shortening
    - hydrogenated and partially hydrogenated oils*
    - coconut oil*
    - palm and palm kernel oils*

*Saturated fats in oil form come from plant sources. Even though they are called "oils," they are considered to be solid fats because they are high in saturated or trans fatty acids.

Monounsaturated Fatty Acid
- A fatty acid that is <u>missing one pair of hydrogen atoms</u> in the middle of the molecule. The gap is called an *unsaturation* and the fatty acid is said to be *monounsaturated* because it has one gap.
- Monounsaturated fatty acids are found mostly in plant food, olive oil, peanut oil, canola oil, avocados, and some types of seafood.
- They tend to lower levels of LDL cholesterol without affecting HDL cholesterol, and they do not promote the formation of artery-clogging fatty deposits.

Polyunsaturated Fatty Acid
- Polyunsaturated fatty acid is a fatty acid that is <u>missing more than one pair of hydrogen atoms</u>.
- Polyunsaturated fatty acids are found mostly in plant food, safflower oil, corn oil, and some types of seafood.
- They tend to lower levels of both HDL cholesterol and LDL cholesterol.
- Polyunsaturated fatty acids do not promote the formation of artery-clogging fatty deposits.
- There are <u>two kinds of polyunsaturated fatty acids</u>:
    - *Omega-3 polyunsaturated fatty acids*
    - *Omega-6 polyunsaturated fatty acids*

4.3.15

Essential Fatty Acids

- **Omega-3 Polyunsaturated Fatty Acid**
- **Omega-6 Polyunsaturated Fatty Acid**
- **Daily Intakes for ALA and LA**
- **Omega-6/Omega-3 Ratio in the Diet**

Fat is essential to the body in order to maintain life. Certain fatty acids that are vital to bodily functions cannot be produced by the body and can only be obtained through one's food intake; these are called essential fatty acids.

There are two kinds of essential fatty acids:

1. Omega-3 polyunsaturated fatty acids
2. Omega-6 polyunsaturated fatty acids

Omega-3 Fatty Acid, or Alpha-Linolenic Acid (LNA or ALA)
- In the body, *alpha-linolenic acid* (LNA) is metabolized to *eicosapentaenoic acid* (EPA) and *docosahexaenoic acid* (DHA).
- Omega-3 fatty acids are found in fish, such as salmon and mackerel, leafy green vegetables, nuts, soybean, canola oil, and especially in flaxseed and flaxseed oil.
- Products available for omega-3 fatty acids are found in a variety of dietary supplements. For example, products containing flaxseed oil provide ALA, fish-oil supplements provide EPA and DHA, and algal oils provide a vegetarian source of DHA.
- Long-term scientific evidence supports the use of omega-3 fatty acids as found in fish oil to reduce sudden death, cardiac death, and myocardial infarction.
- Omega-3 fatty acids lower triglyceride levels in the blood.

Omega-6 Fatty Acid, or Linoleic Acid (LA)
- In the body, *linoleic acid* (LA) is metabolized to *arachidonic acid* (AA).
- Omega-6 fatty acids are found in corn, soybean, and safflower oils.
- Omega-6 fatty acids lower LDL cholesterol levels in the blood.

Daily Intakes for ALA and LA
- The Institute of Medicine has established adequate intakes for ALA and LA (1.1–1.6 grams per day and 11–17 grams per day, respectively, for adults) but not for EPA and DHA.

Omega-6/Omega-3 Ratio in the Diet
- Most American diets provide at least ten times more omega-6 than omega-3 fatty acids. There is now general scientific agreement that individuals should consume more omega-3 and fewer omega-6 fatty acids for good health.
- It is not known, however, whether a desirable ratio of omega-6 to omega-3 fatty acids exists for the diet or to what extent high intakes of omega-6 fatty acids interfere with any benefits of omega-3 fatty acid consumption.

4.3.16

"Bad" Fats

- **Triglycerides**
- **Trans Fatty Acid (or Hydrogenated Fat)**

Triglycerides
- Triglycerides are formed from <u>three fatty acid molecules and one glycerol molecule</u>.
- The main type of naturally occurring fat (lipids) consumed in the diet, triglycerides are found in meats, oils, butter, processed foods, and dairy that is <u>not</u> nonfat.
- Also, the excess calories that we consume, such as carbohydrates, are converted into triglycerides.
- Most of the body's stored fat is in the form of triglycerides, which are transported through the blood to be used by the body's tissues.
- High levels of triglycerides are a risk factor for heart attack or stroke.

Trans Fatty Acid
- Trans fatty acid is formed through an industrial process that adds hydrogen atoms to vegetable oil, and that causes the oil to become solid at room temperature. This chemical process is called *hydrogenation*. The resulting product is a *partially hydrogenated fat,* and it is added to certain processed foods for the purpose of giving them a longer shelf life.
- Some common processed foods that have trans fat (or hydrogenated fats) are baked goods such as cakes, cookies, piecrusts, and crackers, as well as vegetable shortening and some margarines.
- When added to food, trans fatty acid produces a very dangerous product that is a major risk factor for heart attack or stroke. It lowers your HDL ("good") cholesterol, and raises your LDL ("bad") cholesterol.

4.3.17

Dietary Fat Intake

- **Total Fat Intake**
- **Saturated Fat Intake**
- **Cholesterol**

Total Fat Intake
- It is generally recommended to keep your total dietary fat intake to <u>30 percent or less of your total calories consumed.</u> For example, if you consume two thousand calories of food daily, your total fat intake should be six hundred calories or less (30 percent of 2,000 = 600).

Saturated Fat Intake
- Total saturated fat intake should be <u>less than 10 percent of total calories consumed.</u> For example, if you consume two thousand calories of food daily, your total saturated fat intake should be two hundred calories or less (10 percent of 2,000 = 200).

Cholesterol
- If you need to lower your cholesterol, reduce your saturated fat to no more than 5–6 percent of your total daily calories.

The following are very <u>general suggestions</u> for health and weight control. Please discuss them with your doctor before beginning any dietary changes:

- Eat fewer foods of animal origin, such as meat.
- Eat only fat-free or 1-percent low-fat dairy products.
- Eat more plant foods such as fruits, vegetables, and grains.

4.3.18

Vitamins and Minerals

- **Essential Vitamins**
- **Fat-Soluble Vitamins**
- **Water-Soluble Vitamins**
- **Essential Minerals**
- **Macro Minerals**
- **Trace Minerals**

Essential Vitamins

- Vitamins are essential for many vital functions within the body, including normal growth and development, normal metabolism, and for regulating the function of the body's cells.
- The body requires these thirteen vitamins:

    1. Vitamin A   *Retinol*
    2. Vitamin B-1   *Thiamine*
    3. Vitamin B-2   *Riboflavin*
    4. Vitamin B-3   *Niacin*
    5. Vitamin B-5   *Pantothenic Acid*
    6. Vitamin B-6   *Pyridoxine*
    7. Vitamin B-7   *Biotin*
    8. Vitamin B-9   *Folic Acid* (also called Folate)
    9. Vitamin B-12   *Cobalamin*
    10. Vitamin C   *Ascorbic Acid*
    11. Vitamin D   *Cholecalciferol*
    12. Vitamin E   *Alpha-Tocopherol*
    13. Vitamin K   *A type of Phylloquinone*

Fat-Soluble Vitamins
- Vitamins A, D, E, and K, and beta-carotene (which is not actually a vitamin but is converted into vitamin A).
- Any vitamin that is taken in excessive doses may be harmful. The most dangerous of which are vitamins A and D, which are toxic at high dosages.

Water-Soluble Vitamins
- All eight of the B vitamins and vitamin C.
  See a full description for each vitamin in section 4.3.19.

Essential Minerals
- There are more than sixty minerals in the human body. These minerals account for about 4 percent of our body weight.
- However, there are only about twenty-two minerals that are considered essential.
- The following is a list of sixteen of the more familiar minerals found in the body:

1. Boron
2. Calcium
3. Chloride
4. Chromium
5. Copper
6. Fluoride
7. Iodine
8. Iron
9. Magnesium
10. Manganese
11. Molybdenum
12. Phosphorus
13. Potassium
14. Selenium
15. Sodium
16. Zinc

Macro Minerals
- There are seven minerals required by the body in relatively large amounts, from 100 milligrams to 1 gram: calcium, phosphorus, magnesium, sodium, potassium, chloride, and sulfur.

Trace Minerals
- These are minerals that are required by the body in extremely small amounts.
- Examples are copper, iodine, zinc, fluoride, and selenium.

See a full description for each mineral in section 4.3.20.

4.3.19

Vitamin Descriptions

Vitamin A (Retinol)
- Vitamin A helps with vision, bone growth, reproduction, growth of epithelium (cells that line the internal and external surfaces of the body), and fighting infections.
- It is fat-soluble and is found in liver, egg yolks, and whole-milk dairy products from animals and in fish oils.
- It can also be made in the body from a substance found in some fruits and vegetables, such as cantaloupes, carrots, spinach, and sweet potatoes.
- Vitamin A acid (aka all-trans-retinoic acid, ATRA, retinoic acid, or Tretinoin) is made in the body from vitamin A and helps cells to grow and develop, especially in the embryo.
- A form of vitamin A acid made in the laboratory is put on the skin to treat conditions such as acne and is taken by mouth to treat acute promyelocytic leukemia (a fast-growing cancer in which there are too many immature blood-forming cells in the blood and bone marrow).
- Vitamin A and vitamin A acid are being studied in the prevention and treatment of other types of cancer.

Vitamin B-1 (Thiamine)
- A nutrient in the vitamin B complex that helps some enzymes work properly, helps break down sugars in the diet, and keeps nerves and the heart healthy.
- Thiamine is found in pork, organ meats, peas, beans, nuts, and whole grains.
- Vitamin B-1 is water-soluble and must be taken in daily.
- Not enough vitamin B-1 can cause a disease called *beriberi* (a condition marked by heart, nerve, and digestive disorders).
- Too much vitamin B-1 may help cancer cells grow faster.

Vitamin B-2 (Riboflavin)
- A nutrient in the vitamin B complex that helps make red blood cells, helps some enzymes work properly, and keeps skin, nails, and hair healthy.
- Riboflavin is found in milk, eggs, malted barley, organ meats, yeast, and leafy vegetables.
- Vitamin B-2 is water-soluble and must be taken in every day.
- Not enough vitamin B-2 can cause anemia (a low number of red blood cells), mouth sores, and skin problems.
- Amounts of vitamin B-2 may be higher in the blood of patients with some types of cancer.

Vitamin B-3 (Niacin and Nicotinic Acid)
- A nutrient in the vitamin B complex that helps some enzymes work properly and helps skin, nerves, and the digestive tract stay healthy.
- Vitamin B-3 is found in many plant and animal products.
- It is water-soluble and must be taken in every day.
- Not enough vitamin B-3 can cause a disease called *pellagra* (a condition marked by skin, nerve, and digestive disorders).
- A form of vitamin B-3 is being studied in the prevention of skin and other types of cancer. Vitamin B-3 may also help to lower blood cholesterol.

Vitamin B-5 (Pantothenic Acid)
- A nutrient in the vitamin B complex that helps some enzymes use foods to make many substances used in the body and protects cells against damage from peroxides.
- Vitamin B-5 is found in almost all plant and animal foods, is water-soluble, and must be taken in every day.

Vitamin B6 (Pyridoxine)
- A nutrient in the vitamin B complex that helps keep nerves and skin healthy, fights infections, keeps blood sugar levels normal, produces red blood cells, and helps some enzymes work properly.
- Vitamin B-6 is a group of related compounds (pyridoxine, pyridoxal, and pyridoxamine) found in cereals, beans, peas, nuts, meat, poultry, fish, eggs, and bananas. It is water-soluble.
- Not enough vitamin B-6 can cause mouth and tongue sores and nervous disorders.
- Vitamin B-6 is being studied in the prevention of hand-foot syndrome (a disorder caused by certain anticancer drugs and marked by pain, swelling, numbness, tingling, or redness of the hands or feet).

Vitamin B-7 (Biotin)
- A nutrient in the vitamin B complex that helps some enzymes break down substances in the body for energy and helps tissues develop.
- Biotin is found in yeast, whole milk, egg yolks, and organ meats.
- Vitamin B-7 (formerly known as vitamin H) is water-soluble and must be taken in every day.
- Not enough vitamin B-7 can cause skin, nerve, and eye disorders.
- Vitamin B-7 is present in larger amounts in some cancer tissue than in normal tissue. Attaching biotin to substances used to treat some types of cancer helps them find cancer cells.

Vitamin B-9 (Folic Acid or Folate)
- A nutrient in the vitamin B complex that helps to make red blood cells.
- Vitamin B-9 is found in whole-grain breads and cereals, liver, green vegetables, orange juice, lentils, beans, and yeast.
- Folic acid is water-soluble and must be taken in every day.
- Not enough folic acid can cause anemia (a condition in which the number of red blood cells is below normal), diseases of the heart and blood vessels, and defects in the brain and spinal cord in a fetus.
- Folic acid is being studied with vitamin B-12 in the prevention and treatment of cancer.

Vitamin B-12 (Cobalamin and Cyanocobalamin)
- A nutrient in the vitamin B complex that helps make red blood cells, DNA, RNA, energy, and tissues and keeps nerve cells healthy.
- It is found in liver, meat, eggs, poultry, shellfish, milk, and milk products.
- Vitamin B-12 is water-soluble (can dissolve in water) and must be taken in every day.
- Not enough vitamin B-12 can cause certain types of anemia (a condition in which the number of red blood cells is below normal) and neurologic disorders.
- It is being studied with folate in the prevention and treatment of some types of cancer.

Vitamin C (Ascorbic Acid)
- Vitamin C helps fight infections, heal wounds, and keep tissues healthy.
- An antioxidant that helps prevent cell damage caused by free radicals (highly reactive chemicals), vitamin C is found in all fruits and vegetables, especially citrus fruits, strawberries, cantaloupe, green peppers, tomatoes, broccoli, leafy greens, and potatoes.
- Vitamin C is water-soluble and must be taken in every day.
- Vitamin C is being studied in the prevention and treatment of some types of cancer.

Vitamin D (Cholecalciferol)
- Vitamin D helps the body use calcium and phosphorus to make strong bones and teeth.
- It is fat-soluble and is found in fatty fish, egg yolks, and dairy products.
- Not enough vitamin D can cause a bone disease called rickets. It is also being studied in the prevention and treatment of some types of cancer.
- A form of vitamin D that helps the body use calcium and phosphorus to make strong bones and teeth is vitamin D-2, or *ergocalciferol*. It is fat-soluble and is found in plants and yeast.
- Vitamin D-2 is made in the body from vitamin D when the body is exposed to the sun. It is also made in the laboratory and sold as a dietary supplement to help prevent and to treat vitamin D deficiency.
- Vitamin D-3 is yet another form of vitamin D and is better at raising and maintaining required levels of vitamin D in the body.

Vitamin E (Alpha-Tocopherol)
- Vitamin E boosts the immune system and helps keep blood clots from forming. It also helps prevent cell damage caused by free radicals (highly reactive chemicals).
- It is fat-soluble and is found in seeds, nuts, leafy green vegetables, and vegetable oils.
- Vitamin E is being studied in the prevention and treatment of some types of cancer. It is a type of antioxidant.

Vitamin K (K1 & K2)
- Common forms of vitamin K in dietary supplements are *phylloquinone* and *phytonadione* (also called vitamin K1), *menaquinone-4*, and *menaquinone-7* (also called vitamin K2).
- Vitamin K helps to form blood clots and maintain strong bones.
- It is fat-soluble and is found in green leafy vegetables, broccoli, liver, and vegetable oils. Vitamin K is also made by bacteria that live in the large intestine.
- Not enough vitamin K can lead to bleeding and bruising.

4.3.20

Mineral Descriptions

Boron
- Necessary to regulate the body's use of calcium, phosphorus, and magnesium.

Calcium
- Essential for the growth and strength of bones.
- Calcium in the blood stream is used in clotting of the blood, the control of blood pressure, the activation of enzymes, the contraction and relaxation of muscles (including the heart muscle), nerve transmission, and regulation of the passage of body fluids and other materials in and out of tissue cells.
- Ninety-nine percent of the body's calcium is stored in the bones and teeth.
- Vitamin D is vital to the storage of the body's calcium.

Chloride (Chlorine)
- Necessary for regulating fluid in the body, chloride is a component of the hydrochloric acid used by the stomach for the digestion of food.
- Also helps to maintain the acid-base balance of the body.

Chromium
- A mineral that is required in trace amounts, although its mechanisms of action in the body and the amounts needed for optimal health are not well defined.
- Chromium enhances the action of insulin and the storage of carbohydrates, fat, and protein in the body.

Copper
- Necessary for formation of red blood cells, absorption of iron, and bone growth.

Fluoride
- Helps to form bone and teeth and helps to prevent tooth decay.

Iodine
- A mineral found in some foods, especially iodized salt and seafood,
- The body needs iodine to make thyroid hormones. These hormones control the body's metabolism and many other important functions.
- The body also needs thyroid hormones for proper bone and brain development during pregnancy and infancy. Getting enough iodine is important for everyone, especially infants and women who are pregnant.

Iron
- The body uses iron to make *hemoglobin*, a protein in red blood cells that carries oxygen from the lungs to all parts of the body, and *myoglobin*, a protein that provides oxygen to muscles.
- The body also needs iron to make some hormones and connective tissue.

Magnesium
- Magnesium is important for many processes in the body, including regulating muscle and nerve function, blood sugar levels, and blood pressure as well as making protein, bone, and DNA.

Manganese
- An essential component of many body enzymes.
- Necessary for healthy bone development, for production of sex hormones, and for production of carbohydrates and fats.

Molybdenum
- An essential component of many body enzymes.

Phosphorus
- Necessary for development of bones and teeth, and in the body's utilization of carbohydrates, fats, and proteins.

Potassium
- Regulates the balance of fluids in the body as well as helps to regulate the heart, the nervous system, and the kidneys.

Selenium
- Important for reproduction, thyroid gland function, DNA production, and protecting the body from damage caused by free radicals and infection.

Sodium
- Necessary for regulating fluid in the body. Also important for muscle contraction and transmission of nerve impulses.

Zinc
- Located in cells throughout the body, zinc helps the immune system fight off invading bacteria and viruses.
- The body also needs zinc to make proteins and DNA, the genetic material in all cells.
- During pregnancy, infancy, and childhood, the body needs zinc to grow and develop properly.
- Zinc also helps wounds heal and is important for proper senses of taste and smell.

There are more than forty other minerals in the human body that are not listed here.

4.3.21

Free Radicals, Antioxidants, and CoQ10

Free Radicals
- Unstable oxygen molecules that are responsible for a variety of health problems (including cancer, heart problems, cataracts, and speeding up of the aging process), free radicals can build up in cells and cause damage to other molecules, such as DNA, lipids, proteins, and an unknown number of others.
- The damage from free radicals is caused by the process of oxidation during normal metabolism, which results in the destruction of body tissues.
- Oxygen has two atoms that are bound together, and when these oxygen atoms split to form a free radical they become unstable. This unstable oxygen molecule has only a single electron.

Antioxidants
- Substances that protect cells from damage caused by free radicals.
- Examples of antioxidants are beta-carotene, lycopene, vitamins A, C, and E, and other natural and manufactured substances.
- The body also produces certain enzymes and compounds that act as antioxidants.

See CoQ10 on the next page.

CoQ10 (coenzyme Q10, Q10, ubiquinone, and vitamin Q-10)
- Coenzyme Q10 (CoQ10) is an antioxidant that is necessary for cells to function properly.
- It is found in plants, bacteria, animals, and people.
- Cells use CoQ10 to make the energy they need to grow and stay healthy.
- CoQ10 can be found in highest amounts in the heart, liver, kidneys, and pancreas.
- Fish, meats, and whole grains all have small amounts of CoQ10, but not enough to significantly boost the levels in your body.
- A variety of diseases, including some genetic disorders, are associated with low levels of CoQ10
- Levels of CoQ10 decrease as you age.
- CoQ10 supplements may benefit some patients with cardiovascular disorders.
- Researchers have also looked at the effects of CoQ10 for drug-induced muscle weakness, reproductive disorders, cancer, and other diseases. However, results from these studies are limited and not conclusive.

4.3.22

Phytochemicals (Plant Chemicals)

- Certain phytochemicals are highly beneficial because they act as antioxidants by disposing of harmful free radicals. They also are believed to offer protection against heart disease and inhibit macular degeneration, which can cause blindness.

- About four thousand phytochemicals have already been identified, and we know there are countless others that have not yet been discovered.

- They have no nutritional value, they are not vitamins or minerals, and they don't even have any calories. Nobody knows what amounts the body requires.

- Another benefit of phytochemicals is that they add the taste, smell, and color to fruits and vegetables.

- Some examples of foods that contain phytochemicals are berries, chili peppers, garlic, onions, broccoli, kale, cabbage, seeds, grapes, tomatoes, soy, orange and yellow fruits and vegetables, green leafy vegetables, nuts, whole grains, rosemary, ginger, oregano, and tea (green, black, or oolong, but <u>not</u> herbal tea).

CHAPTER 5

The Circulatory System

5.1 Anatomy of the Circulatory System ·············· 233
    5.1.1   Components of the Circulatory System ·············· 235
    5.1.2   Heart ·············· 237
    5.1.3   Structure of the Heart ·············· 239
    5.1.4   Layers of the Heart Wall ·············· 240
    5.1.5   Heart Chambers ·············· 241
    5.1.6   The Heart Map ·············· 243
    5.1.7   Diagnosing Circulatory Sounds ·············· 245
    5.1.8   Blood Pressure ·············· 247
    5.1.9   Pulse ·············· 248
    5.1.10 Cardio Measurements ·············· 249
    5.1.11 Blood Function ·············· 251
    5.1.12 Blood Components ·············· 252
    5.1.13 Types of Blood Vessels ·············· 254
    5.1.14 Circulatory System - Image ·············· 258

5.2 Heart Healthy Exercise ·············· 259
    5.2.1   Ergometer ·············· 261
    5.2.2   Cardio Endurance ·············· 262
    5.2.3   The Capacity to Consume Oxygen ·············· 263
    5.2.4   Aerobic Training Guidelines (Beginners) ·············· 264
    5.2.5   MET System ·············· 271
    5.2.6   Maximum Heart Rate and Calculations ·············· 273
    5.2.7   Maximum Heart Rate Compared to Aerobic Capacity ·············· 275
    5.2.8   Karvonen Formula ·············· 276
    5.2.9   Karvonen Formula Calculations ·············· 277
    5.2.10 Using the Karvonen Formula ·············· 278
    5.2.11 How to Train Safely ·············· 280

5.3 Circulatory System Injuries and Conditions ·····················283
    5.3.1   Heart Conditions ··285
    5.3.2   Blood Conditions··288
    5.3.3   Understanding Cholesterol ·································289
    5.3.4   Cholesterol Terms ··290
    5.3.5   Cholesterol Range References ·····························292
    5.3.6   Dietary Fat and Cholesterol Levels·······················293
    5.3.7   Blood Vessel Conditions ·····································295

5.1 Anatomy of the Circulatory System

5.1.1

Components of the Circulatory System

- **Heart**
- **Lungs**
- **Blood Vessels**

- The **cardiovascular** and **cardiopulmonary** systems work to distribute oxygen and nutrients throughout the body. This system also helps to remove carbon dioxide and other metabolic waste from the cells of the body.

- In addition to these main functions, these systems also help to control body temperature, form blood clots to prevent excessive bleeding, and protect the body against disease.

Here is how the three main parts of the systems work together:

Part # 1: Heart
- The heart is the pumping mechanism that provides for the <u>blood circulation cycle throughout the body</u>. Every system of the body requires oxygenated blood, <u>including the heart</u>.
- Blood will leave the heart oxygenated and return to it deoxygenated.

Part # 2: Lungs
- The lungs receive deoxygenated blood and reoxygenate it for another cycle through the body.
- **See Chapter 6: The Respiratory System.**

Part # 3: Blood Vessels
- <u>Arteries</u> are the vessels that carry <u>oxygenated</u> blood from the heart to all the body's tissues.
- As this blood is continuously being used by the body's tissues, it becomes increasingly depleted of oxygen.
- <u>Veins</u> then carry this mostly <u>deoxygenated</u> blood back to the heart and lungs where it will again be oxygenated.
- This cycle is continuous as the arteries will again carry this freshly oxygenated blood back out to all the body's tissues.

See section 5.1.13 for Types of Blood Vessels.

5.1.2

Heart

Anatomy of the Human Heart

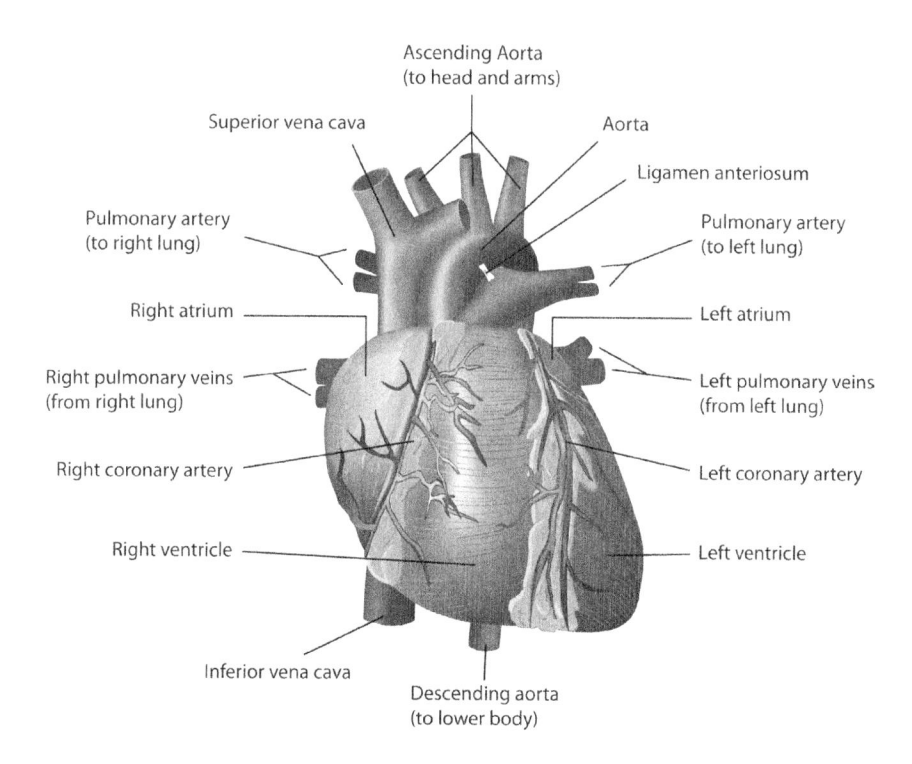

- Ascending Aorta (to head and arms)
- Superior vena cava
- Aorta
- Ligamen anteriosum
- Pulmonary artery (to right lung)
- Pulmonary artery (to left lung)
- Right atrium
- Left atrium
- Right pulmonary veins (from right lung)
- Left pulmonary veins (from left lung)
- Right coronary artery
- Left coronary artery
- Right ventricle
- Left ventricle
- Inferior vena cava
- Descending aorta (to lower body)

- The heart is a muscular pump that provides the force necessary to circulate the blood to all the tissues in the body.

- Its function is vital because tissues need a continuous supply of oxygen and nutrients to survive, and metabolic waste products have to be removed. Deprived of these necessities, cells soon undergo irreversible changes that lead to death.

- While blood is the transport medium, the heart is the organ that keeps the blood moving through the vessels.

- An electrical system controls the heart and uses electrical signals to contract the heart's walls. When the walls contract, blood is pumped into the circulatory system. Inlet and outlet valves in the heart chambers ensure that blood flows in the right direction.

- The normal adult heart pumps about five liters of blood every minute.

- If the heart loses its pumping effectiveness for even a few minutes, the individual's life is jeopardized.

5.1.3

Structure of the Heart

- The human heart is a four-chambered muscular organ, shaped and sized roughly like a closed fist with two-thirds of the mass to the left of midline.

- The heart is enclosed in the *pericardium*, a double-walled sac containing the heart and the roots of the *great vessels*.

- The <u>great vessels</u> are the large vessels that bring blood to and from the heart: *superior vena cava, inferior vena cava, pulmonary arteries, pulmonary veins*, and *aorta*.

- The *pericardium* attaches the heart to the *mediastinum* (the central compartment of the thoracic cavity surrounded by loose connective tissue), gives protection against infection, and provides the lubrication for the heart.

5.1.4

Layers of the Heart Wall

- **Epicardium**
- **Myocardium**
- **Endocardium**

Three layers of tissue form the heart wall. The <u>outer layer</u> is the *epicardium*, the <u>middle layer</u> is the *myocardium*, and the <u>inner layer</u> is the *endocardium*.

Epicardium
- The epicardium is the smooth outer membrane of the heart that is primarily composed of connective tissue and functions as a protective layer.

Myocardium
- The myocardium is the heart muscle and is also referred to as the muscular wall of the heart.
- Its muscle tissue is composed of striated involuntary muscle cells (*myocytes* and *cardiac*) that are connected and form the contractile pump that generates the hearts blood flow.
- *Myocytes* are the muscle cells that make up the cardiac muscle.

Endocardium
- The endocardium is the innermost layer of tissue that lines the chambers of the heart.
- Its cells are embryologically and biologically similar to the endothelial cells that line blood vessels.
- The endocardium also provides protection to the valves and heart chambers.

5.1.5

Heart Chambers

- **Upper Chambers**
- **Lower Chambers**
- **Circulation of Blood**

The heart is the epicenter of the cardiovascular system, and it is divided into four separate chambers:

Upper Chambers
1. Right atrium: receives deoxygenated blood from all parts of the body, except from the lungs.
2. Left atrium: receives oxygenated blood from the lungs.

Lower Chambers
1. Right ventricle: pumps deoxygenated blood to the lungs.
2. Left ventricle: pumps oxygenated blood throughout the body, except into the lungs.

Circulation of Blood Through the Heart

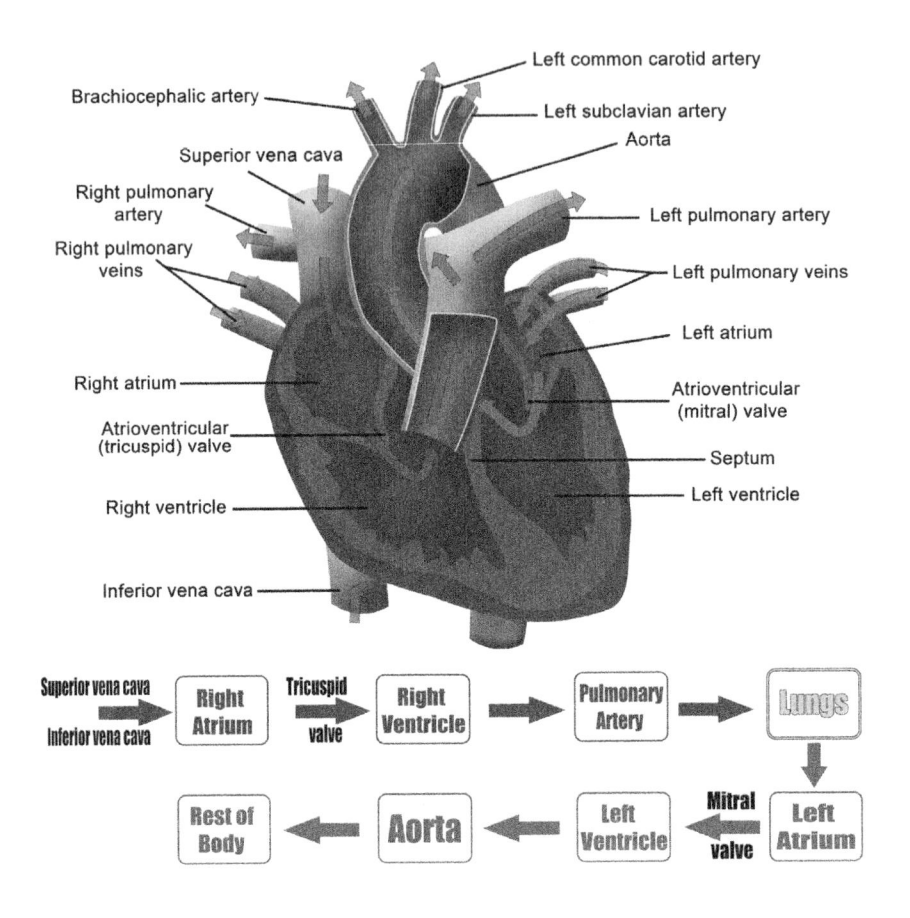

5.1.6

The Heart Map

The Heart Map explains the:
- functional interaction between the heart and lungs
- circulation pathways of the blood through the heart and lungs
- names of the heart chambers
- blood oxygen level as it is received or exits each chamber

Quick Overview
1. The heart receives the deoxygenated blood and pumps it into the lungs to get oxygenated.
2. After oxygenation occurs in the lungs, the oxygenated blood is pumped back into the heart.
3. The heart then pumps out the newly oxygenated blood to be circulated throughout the body and all of its tissues.

More Detailed Map
1. After the blood has circulated throughout the body, it returns to the heart almost totally depleted of oxygen.
2. This deoxygenated blood enters the heart through the vena cava.
3. From the vena cava, the deoxygenated blood enters into the right atrium.
4. From the right atrium, the deoxygenated blood goes to the right ventricle.
5. From the right ventricle, the deoxygenated blood goes into the lungs.
6. In the lungs, the deoxygenated blood becomes oxygenated.
7. From the lungs, the oxygenated blood goes to the left atrium.
8. From the left atrium, the oxygenated blood goes to the left ventricle.
9. From the left ventricle, the freshly oxygenated blood is then pumped out of the heart and circulated throughout the body to replenish all the body's cells.

5.1.7

Diagnosing Circulatory Sounds

- **Stethoscope**
- **Sphygmomanometer**
- **Auscultation**
- **Korotkoff Sounds**

Stethoscope
- A device used to listen to internal body sounds, such as the heartbeat as well as the passage of air through the lungs and sounds in the abdominal region.

Sphygmomanometer
- A device, along with a stethoscope, that is used to measure blood pressure.
- The sphygmomanometer is comprised of a rubber bladder that is enclosed in a nylon cuff and connected to an inflating bulb.
- The blood pressure is read on the manometer.

Auscultation
- Listening to bodily sounds by using a stethoscope.
- The most familiar uses are to listen to the heartbeat, lungs, and the sounds that are used to measure blood pressure.
- Auscultation is also used for the purpose of listening to other sounds from within the body that are necessary to make a diagnosis.

Korotkoff Sounds
- With the use of a sphygmomanometer, these are the sounds used to determine blood pressure.
- There are <u>five different sounds</u> as the blood pulsates through the brachial artery. Each of these sounds are referred to as a *phase*:

    Phase I: The appearance of clear tapping sounds.
    Phase II: The sounds become softer and longer.
    Phase III: The sounds become crisper and louder.
    Phase IV: The sounds become muffled and softer.
    Phase V: The sounds disappear.

- It is necessary to <u>distinguish</u> the sounds in order to determine blood pressure.
- **Phases I & V** represent the <u>*systolic* blood pressure</u>, and the <u>*diastolic* blood pressure</u>, respectively.

5.1.8

Blood Pressure

- **Systolic Blood Pressure**
- **Diastolic Blood Pressure**
- **High Blood Pressure (Hypertension)**
- **Essential Hypertension**
- **White Coat Hypertension**

Systolic Blood Pressure
- The pressure exerted by the blood on the blood vessel walls with each heartbeat.

Diastolic Blood Pressure
- The pressure exerted by the blood on the blood vessel walls when the heart rests between beats.

<u>Normal blood pressure is 120 systolic over 80 diastolic, or 120/80.</u>

High Blood Pressure, or Hypertension
- Interchangeable terms that apply when blood pressure is greater than <u>140 systolic over 90 diastolic,</u> or 140/90.

Essential Hypertension
- More than 90 percent of all high blood pressure (hypertension) has no known cause and is referred to as essential hypertension.

White Coat Hypertension
- An increase in blood pressure that only occurs when a person goes to the doctor. This temporary elevation in blood pressure is related to anxiety and not to the condition of hypertension.

5.1.9

Pulse

- **Palpation**
- **Carotid Pulse Site**
- **Radial Pulse Site**
- **Temporal Pulse Site**
- **Apical Pulse Site**

Pulse
- The rhythmic expansion and contraction of an artery caused by blood being forced through it by the pumping action of the heart.

Palpation
- The use of fingers at a pulse site to measure the pulse rate.

Carotid Pulse Site
- Located on each side of the front of the neck, over the *carotid arteries*, just below the angle of the jaw.

Radial Pulse Site
- Located on the wrists, over the *radial arteries*, just under the thumb.

Temporal Pulse Site
- Located on each side of the head, on the temple directly in front of the ear, over the *superficial temporal arteries* and extended from the carotid arteries.

Apical Pulse Site
- Located over the *apex of the heart*, at the lower left of the heart, and its sounds are heard through a stethoscope.

5.1.10

Cardio Measurements

- **Heart Rate**
- **Resting Heart Rate**
- **Cardiac Output**
- **Stroke Volume**
- **Ejection Fraction**
- **Oxygen Extraction**

Heart Rate (HR)
- The number of times the heart beats each minute, also referred to as *beats per minute* or bpm.

Resting Heart Rate (RHR)
- The number of times the heart beats each minute when a person is completely at rest.
- The resting heart rate can only be determined after a person has rested quietly for at least four or five minutes, either sitting or lying down.
- The average resting heart rate is about seventy-two beats per minute.

Cardiac Output
- The amount of blood pumped by the heart <u>each minute</u>.
- The average heart pumps about one gallon of blood each minute.

Stroke Volume
- The amount of blood pumped by each ventricle <u>each time the heart beats</u>.

Ejection Fraction
- The percentage of the total volume of blood in the ventricles that is pumped out each time the heart beats.
- The amount of blood that fills the ventricles during the rest period between heartbeats is not always completely pumped out during a heartbeat.
- At rest the ejection fraction is only about 50 percent, and during exercise the ejection fraction can increase up to 100 percent.

Oxygen Extraction
- The process wherein oxygen is removed from the blood to be used by the muscles.
- This removal of oxygen takes place in the capillaries of the muscles.

5.1.11

Blood Function

- Blood acts as the body's transport system and it has the ability to prevent its own loss by clotting. Adults have about ten pints.

- With a resting heart rate, the heart pumps about ten pints per minute throughout the body. During exercise the heart may pump forty pints or more a minute.

- Approximately half of the volume of our blood is made of cells. There are red cells (*erythrocytes*), white cells (*leukocytes*), and platelets (*thrombocytes*). The remaining volume of blood is called *plasma* (see next section).

- One of the main functions of the blood is that its red blood cells contain the protein hemoglobin, which transports oxygen throughout the body.

- Another important function of the blood is that its white blood cells have the ability to defend against viruses, bacteria, fungi, and parasites and therefore help to establish our immune system.

- Blood stops bleeding (also referred to as *clotting*) and helps in the repair of damaged blood vessels. The substance in blood that performs these two functions is called *platelets* (see next section).

5.1.12

Blood Components

- **Platelets**
- **Plasma**
- **Hemoglobin**
- **Red Blood Cells**
- **White Blood Cells**

Platelets
- Platelets are cells that circulate in our blood.
- When a person gets a cut or sustains an injury, these platelets bind together at the site of the damaged blood vessel and cause the blood to clot, which stops the bleeding.
- Platelets are created in the bone marrow, the same area for the production of red blood cells, and most of the white blood cells.

Plasma
- Another important component of blood is plasma, which is about 95 percent water. It also contains salt, proteins, sugars, fats, and minerals.
- Plasma serves many functions such as carrying nutrients throughout the body. It also carries away waste products, such as urea.
- Additionally, each gland manufactures its own unique hormone to be used specifically for its intended organ. Plasma carries these hormones to their intended destinations.

Hemoglobin
- A protein in red blood cells that contains iron, carries oxygen throughout the body, and is responsible for the red color of blood.

Red Blood Cells (*Erythrocytes*)
- The body's most common type of blood cells and the primary method for transporting oxygen throughout the body.
- Red blood cells also transport carbon dioxide to the lungs for removal when you exhale.
- These cells also contain a protein called hemoglobin, described above.

White Blood Cells (*Leukocytes*)
- A major component of our immune system, white blood cells help to defend the body against infection by protecting against disease.
- All white blood cells are produced in the bone marrow.

5.1.13

Types of Blood Vessels

Arteries

- Arteries
- Aorta
- Coronary Arteries
- Carotid Artery
- Arterioles
- Capillaries
- Pulmonary Arteries

Veins

- Venous System
- Vena Cava
- Veins
- Venules
- Pulmonary Veins
- Vascular
- Avascular
- Therapeutic - Angiogenesis

Artery and Vein

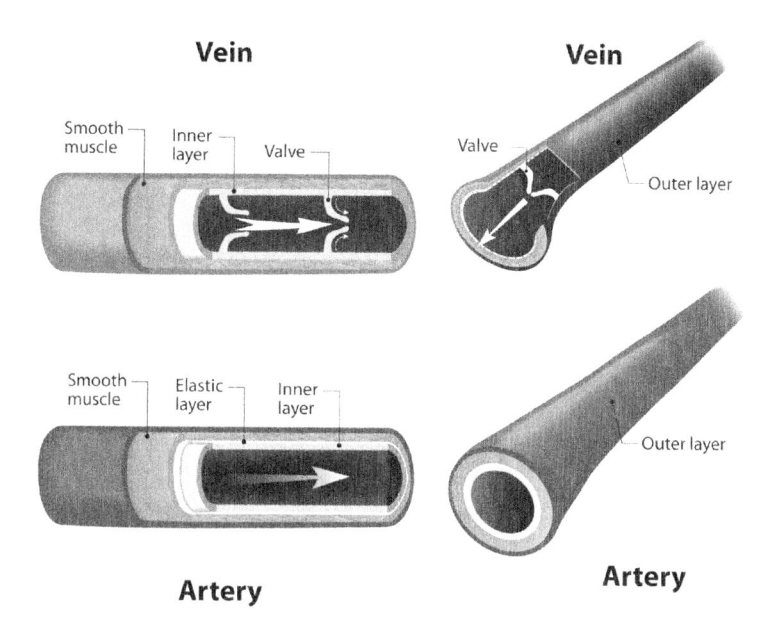

Arteries
- The largest blood vessels in the body. They carry oxygen-rich blood away from the heart to nourish all the tissues of the body.
- Arteries have muscular walls that help them push the blood throughout the body. They are much stronger than veins.

Aorta
- The largest artery in the body, the aorta receives freshly oxygenated blood from the lungs via the muscular left ventricle of the heart, and then pumps that blood out to the entire body.

Coronary Arteries
- The two vessels originating from the aorta that supply all parts of the heart muscle with oxygen-rich blood.

Carotid Arteries
- The main arteries that are located on each side of the neck, one on each side. They are one of the easiest places to feel a pulse.

Arterioles
- As <u>arteries get further from the heart</u>, their sizes becomes smaller, and these smaller arteries are referred to as arterioles.

Capillaries
- As the <u>arterioles get even further from the heart</u>, they become the smallest blood vessels (*capillaries*) that can carry oxygen-rich blood to the tissues of the body.

Pulmonary Arteries
- <u>The arteries that deliver deoxygenated blood from the heart to the lungs</u>. They differ from the other major arteries whose purpose is to deliver oxygenated blood from the heart to the body's tissues.
- The main pulmonary artery comes out of the right ventricle of the heart and divides into the right and left pulmonary arteries, which enter into the right and left lungs.

Venous System
- This entire network of blood vessels consists of the veins. They carry blood that is depleted in oxygen, and higher in carbon dioxide, back to the heart.

Vena Cava
- Two very large veins that receive deoxygenated blood from the body and return it to the right atrium of the heart.
- The superior (<u>upper</u>) vena cava collects blood from the <u>upper parts of the body,</u> such as the head, neck, and arms.
- The inferior (<u>lower</u>) vena cava collects blood from the <u>lower parts of the body,</u> such as the legs and abdomen area.

Veins
- Any of a series of blood vessels from throughout the body that carry deoxygenated blood back to the heart.
- Veins have valves to prevent blood from flowing backward.
- Blood collected by the veins is somewhat higher in carbon dioxide than freshly oxygenated blood.

Venules
- The thinner divisions of the veins.

Pulmonary Veins
- These veins deliver **oxygenated** blood from the lungs to the left atrium of the heart.
- They differ from the other veins whose purpose is to deliver **deoxygenated blood** to the heart.
    - The four pulmonary veins are:
        1. the right superior
        2. right inferior
        3. left superior
        4. left inferior

Vascular
- A term that refers to blood vessels, or to a blood vessel system that also carries body fluids such as lymph throughout the body.

Avascular
- A term indicating the existence of few or no blood vessels in a body system.

Therapeutic Angiogenesis
- The use of genes to grow new blood vessels to repair or replace damaged blood vessels in the heart muscle.

5.1.14

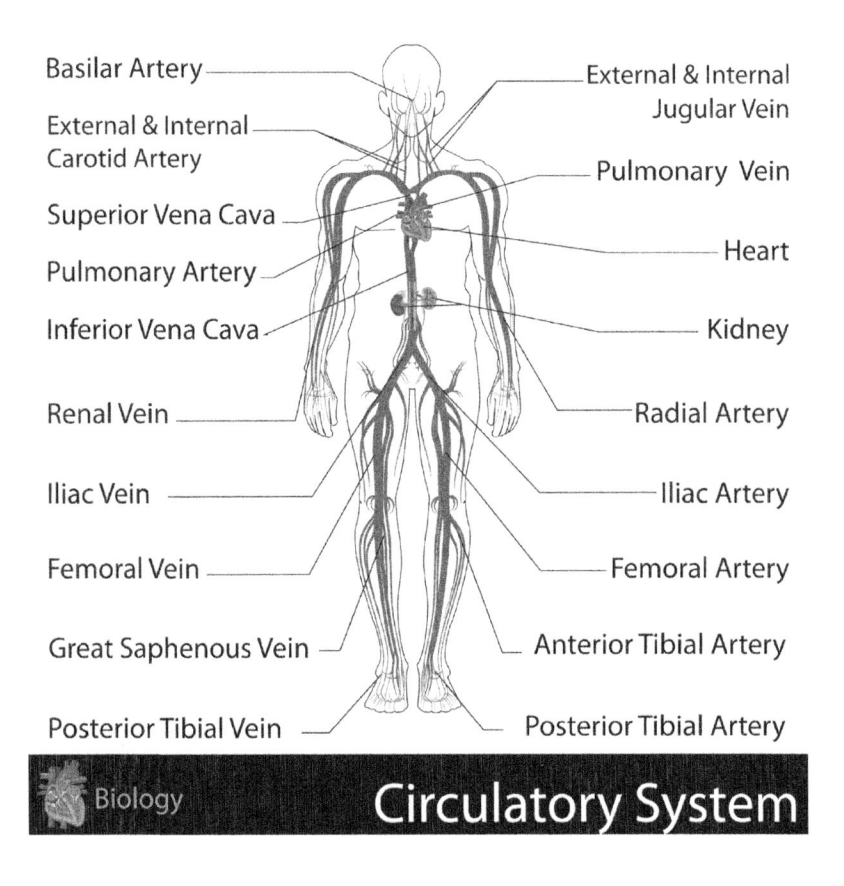

Basilar Artery	External & Internal Jugular Vein
External & Internal Carotid Artery	Pulmonary Vein
Superior Vena Cava	Heart
Pulmonary Artery	
Inferior Vena Cava	Kidney
Renal Vein	Radial Artery
Iliac Vein	Iliac Artery
Femoral Vein	Femoral Artery
Great Saphenous Vein	Anterior Tibial Artery
Posterior Tibial Vein	Posterior Tibial Artery

Biology **Circulatory System**

5.2 Heart Healthy Exercise

5.2.1

Ergometer

- Used to continuously measure and record both the <u>amount of physical work done by the body</u> and also the <u>body's response to that work</u>. The amount of physical work to be done is predetermined.

- The device continuously measures and records heart function, such as heart rate and heart rhythm as well as blood pressure.

- It also measures and records the breathing rate and the volume of oxygen that is consumed.

- Ergometers can be stationary bicycles, treadmills, or rowing machines and are primarily used for fitness and stress testing.

5.2.2

Cardio Endurance

- **Cardiovascular Endurance**
- **Cardiopulmonary Endurance**
- **Cardiorespiratory Endurance**

These three exercise terms, typically used interchangeably, relate to the ability of the heart and lungs to deliver enough oxygenated blood to the large muscles so that they can produce the energy necessary for sustained motion.

5.2.3

The Capacity to Consume Oxygen

- **VO2 Max**
- **Max Cardiac Output**
- **Max Oxygen Extraction**

These three technical terms are collectively known as <u>the capacity to consume oxygen</u>, which refers to the highest volume of oxygen that a person can consume during aerobic exercise.

VO2 Max
- Max Cardiac Output x Max Oxygen Extraction
- The most desirable intensity range for VO2 Max is 50–85 percent.

Max Cardiac Output
- The amount of blood pumped by the heart each minute. The average heart pumps about one gallon of blood each minute.

Max Oxygen Extraction
- The process wherein oxygen is removed from the blood to be used by the muscles. This removal of oxygen takes place in the capillaries of the muscles.
- A *graded exercise stress test* is used to determine a person's precise maximum aerobic capacity.

5.2.4

Aerobic Training Guidelines (Beginners)

- Intensity
- Frequency
- Duration
- Warm-Up
- Stretch
- Training Heart Rate Chart
- Aerobic Conditioning Exercise Program
- Aerobic Conditioning Progression Plan
- Initial Conditioning Stage
- Improvement Conditioning Stage
- Maintenance Conditioning Stage
- Cardiorespiratory Training Methods:
  - Continuous Training
  - Interval Training
  - Fartlek Training
  - Circuit Training
  - Aerobic Composite Training
- Cool-Down

Intensity
- The effort required to perform an aerobic exercise.
- When using the Training Heart Rate Chart to calculate intensity, it should be the effort that falls within 60–90 percent of this chart.
- In order to condition your heart, you must bring your heart rate up to an appropriate level and continue for an appropriate amount of time based on your level of fitness.

Frequency
- How often an aerobic exercise is performed.
- If you are a beginner, it is recommended that you start exercising at least three times per week.
- Gradually increase exercising to five to six times per week.

Duration
- The time required to perform an aerobic exercise.
- If you are a beginner, it is recommended that you start with fifteen to twenty minutes of exercise per workout.
- Gradually increase to thirty minutes of exercise per workout.

Warm-Up
- An aerobic warm-up should last from five to eight minutes, using the same muscles that will be used for the planned aerobic activity.

Stretch
- Be sure to stretch the same muscles that will be used for the planned aerobic activity.

Training Heart Rate Chart

Ideal training heart rate is

60–75 percent of maximum heart rate (MHR)

Age	Training HR	MHR
20	120–150 bpm	200 bpm
25	117–146 bpm	195 bpm
30	114–142 bpm	190 bpm
35	111–138 bpm	185 bpm
40	108–135 bpm	180 bpm
45	105–131 bpm	175 bpm
50	102–127 bpm	170 bpm
55	99–123 bpm	165 bpm
60	96–120 bpm	160 bpm
65	93–116 bpm	155 bpm
70	90–113 bpm	150 bpm

Aerobic Conditioning Exercise Program
- The components of an <u>aerobic conditioning exercise program</u> must include a plan for the following:
    - fitness goals
    - endurance objectives *(strength objectives would be part of an <u>anaerobic</u> program)*
    - a warm-up and cool-down
    - selection of the type of exercise
    - frequency of the exercise
    - duration of the exercise
    - intensity of the exercise
    - flexibility training
    - a progression plan
    - safety awareness

Aerobic Conditioning Progression Plan
- Periodically, certain components of the exercise program must be reevaluated to assure that the program reflects improvement.
- As an individual progresses, particular emphasis should be applied to increasing:
    - frequency of the exercise
    - duration of the exercise
    - intensity of the exercise
    - level of flexibility

Initial Conditioning Stage
- This first stage is where the body prepares for an aerobic conditioning program and it lasts for approximately four to six weeks.
- It is suggested that a person in the initial conditioning stage use a beginner's level in the following:
    - aerobic exercises
    - stretching
    - calisthenics
- In the beginning, the exercise frequency should be every other day.
- The exercise duration (time) should be between twelve and fifteen minutes.
- Note that the intensity level of normal aerobic exercise programs is within 60–90 percent of the maximum heart rate.
- However, in the initial conditioning stage, it is recommended that a beginner start exercising conservatively at a maximum heart rate level close to the 60 percent range.
- This intensity may vary according to such factors as:
    - age
    - level of fitness
    - bodyweight
    - medical condition or numerous other factors
- It is recommended that people over the age of fifty get the approval of their physician to begin a planned exercise program.
- Approval is also recommended for people of any age who have health conditions.

Improvement Conditioning Stage
- This second stage is where most of the aerobic conditioning occurs and it lasts for approximately eight to twenty weeks.
- Exercise intensity, and duration increase more rapidly than in the initial conditioning stage.
- Frequency is increased to five times per week.

Maintenance Conditioning Stage
- This third stage is where a person has met her fitness goals and seeks to maintain them.
- Periodic reevaluation is recommended.
- Exercise variations are helpful to ward off boredom and to maximize the effects of one's exercise routine.
- Frequency may be increased to six times per week for the advanced exerciser.

Cardiorespiratory Training Methods
- There are five basic types of cardiorespiratory training:
    1. Continuous Training
    2. Interval Training
    3. Fartlek Training
    4. Circuit Training
    5. Aerobic Composite Training

1. **Continuous Training**
    - A method of training that maintains the level of intensity between 50–85 percent of maximal oxygen consumption.
    - Continuous training is divided into two categories:
        1. *Intermediate slow distance,* which is continuous aerobic exercise for a period of twenty to sixty minutes.
        2. *Long slow distance,* which is continuous aerobic exercise for a period of more than sixty minutes.

2. **Interval Training**
    - A method of training that uses high levels of intensity interspersed with low levels of intensity in repeated intervals.
    - This type of training is especially beneficial for people who are just beginning an aerobic exercise program or those who have a low cardiorespiratory classification. The reason is that it gives the individual an opportunity to recover during the low-level intensity spurts that are part of interval training.
    - An example of interval training is bicycling for three minutes at a high intensity, immediately followed by two minutes at very low intensity.
    - This changeover can be repeated five to ten times in a workout session.
    - The number of times a person would <u>repeat</u> this method of switching from high level intensity to low-level intensity is determined by the level of fitness of the individual.
    - Also, the level of <u>intensity</u> used both at the upper end and the lower end is determined by the level of fitness of the individual.

3. **Fartlek Training**
    - A form of training similar to interval training.
    - High intensity–low intensity intervals are not specifically measured, but instead are determined by how the participant feels.

4. **Circuit Training**
    - Strength training using approximately ten to twelve exercise machines that are designed to train the major muscle groups going in order from the larger muscle groups to the smaller muscle groups.
    - It is a time-efficient method that usually takes about twenty to twenty-five minutes and performed in rapid succession, adding some level of aerobic conditioning as well.

5. **Aerobic Cross Training (Aerobic Composite Training)**
    - An individualized aerobic training preference that is useful in overcoming boredom and overtraining.
    - Individuals use any variety of training methods, as well as any variety of intensities or aerobic training devices.
    - Generally done by individuals who are in the maintenance phase of conditioning.
    - Training variations are unlimited and spontaneous, and an individual may alternate between two or more aerobic activities at different levels of intensity and with some discretion.
    - The changeover from one exercise to another helps to prevent overtraining to a particular muscle group and gives the body a more thorough muscular workout along with the aerobic benefits.
    - A typical example of a fifty-minute aerobic cross training workout is warming up by jogging for fifteen minutes, then riding a bicycle at a high intensity for twenty minutes, and then gradually cooling down on a treadmill for another fifteen minutes.

Cool-Down
- To reduce bodily risk after your work out, it is essential that you cool down your body for at least five to ten minutes by <u>performing low level aerobic exercise</u>.
- You can use any aerobic exercise machine, but gradually taper the intensity so that when you finish, your aerobic effort is equivalent to a very slow walk.

Benefits:
- Reduces the possibility of blood pooling, a sudden drop in blood pressure, lightheadedness, dizziness, and fainting.
- Reduces the possibility of muscle spasms and cramping.
- Reduces the amounts of beneficial hormones such as endorphins that are produced from vigorous exercise.
- It is very important to lower the amounts of these hormones to reduce the risk of cardiac rhythm irregularities.

5.2.5

MET System

- **Rate of Perceived Exertion**
- **Talk Test**

- The intensity of an exercise may be designed to conform to a desired percentage (between 50–85 percent) of an exerciser's maximum oxygen consumption, which can also be described as the functional oxygen capacity (or VO2 max).
- This is a technical system that classifies physical activities by metabolic equivalents, known as METs. One MET is equivalent to a person's oxygen consumption at rest. This amount is about 3.5 milliliters of oxygen per kilogram of body weight per minute (3.5 ml/kg/min).
- The amount of time a person stays on the bicycle or treadmill makes it possible to estimate and convert the maximum oxygen consumption to a MET equivalent.
- The MET system is used to measure exercise intensity for any sports activity and to derive an approximate energy measurement for those sports activities.
- Furthermore, the necessary data derived from stress tests may be described in MET values.

Rate of Perceived Exertion (A Scale to Assess Exertion)

- This exertion scale was designed by Dr. Gunnar Borg and is often referred to as the Borg Scale.
- It assigns subjective numerical values that are used to perceive the rate of exertion. On the Borg Scale, the range is from six to twenty. As an example, a perceived rate of six indicates no exertion. A perceived rate of thirteen would indicate a more difficult rate of exertion, and a perceived rate of twenty would indicate maximal exertion.
- Recently a new rating scale has been developed, and the numerical values are different. This new scale has a range from zero to ten. As an example, a perceived rate of zero indicates no exertion. A perceived rate of four would indicate a somewhat difficult rate of exertion. A perceived rate of ten would indicate maximal exertion.

Talk Test
- By observing the required effort to breathe and the required effort to talk during exercise, a subjective level of exertion can be determined.
- This method is very helpful in determining a safety zone for aerobic activity.
- To maintain this safety zone, exercisers should keep the intensity of the exercise at a level that enables them to speak and breathe with relative ease.

5.2.6

Maximum Heart Rate and Calculations

- Maximum Heart Rate (MHR)
- Training Heart Rate Range (THRR)

Maximum Heart Rate (MHR) Formula
- MHR = 220 bpm – age

Training Heart Rate Range (THRR)
- The accepted intensities for aerobic training. They should be between 60–90 percent of a person's maximum heart rate (MHR), and are calculated to determine both the upper and lower age-related training heart rate.

- Using the MHR formula is one of the safest ways to monitor a training program. People interested in fat loss should begin a program between 60–75 percent of their MHR.

- In any aerobics exercise program, it is recommended that you consult a certified personal fitness trainer to determine your THRR. Many gyms have charts to assist in determining the appropriate range of intensity for each age group.

Calculations for Lower and Upper Limits of MHR:
- Lower Limit = MHR x 60 percent
- Upper Limit = MHR x 75 percent

Calculation Example:
- A fifty-year-old adult wants to train at the suggested rates of 60–75 percent of his maximum heart rate.
- MHR = 220 bpm – age = (220 – 50) = 170
- Lower limit is 170 x 60 percent = 102
- Upper limit is 170 x 75 percent = 128
- Therefore, the THRR for this fifty-year-old is between 102 and 128 beats per minute.

5.2.7

Maximum Heart Rate Compared to Aerobic Capacity

For comparison, it is necessary to know the relationship between <u>maximum heart rate</u> (60–90 percent) and <u>aerobic capacity/maximum oxygen consumption</u> (50–85 percent).

At almost all levels of <u>submaximal aerobic exercise</u>, the percentage of maximum heart rate *does not equal* the same percentage of aerobic capacity unless the <u>Karvonen Formula</u> (also known as the Heart Rate Maximum Reserve Method) is used.

- Learn about the Karvonen Formula in the following section.

5.2.8

Karvonen Formula

- One of the most popular methods for calculating exercise heart rates.

- It is a more accurate method than the maximum heart rate for finding the training heart rate range for an individual wishing to perform aerobic exercises.

- Though the Karvonen Formula is similar to the maximum heart rate method, it is not the same because resting heart rate (RHR) is calculated into the formula.

5.2.9

Karvonen Formula Calculations

Abbreviations used for the Karvonen Formula Calculations

(Also used in other aerobic calculations)

- MHR (Maximum Heart Rate) = (220 – age)
- Workout Intensity = ideally 60–90 percent of MHR
- RHR (Resting Heart Rate) = an average of 72 bpm
- HRR (Heart Rate Reserve) = the MHR – RHR
- Aerobic Workout Intensity = ideally 50–85 percent of MHR
- THR (Training Heart Rate) = HRR x Aerobic Intensity + RHR

The desired intensities for the Karvonen Formula must always be between 50–85 percent.

5.2.10

Using the Karvonen Formula

Example
- **To use the Karvonen Formula to calculate a desired training heart rate, let's assume:**
    - the person is fifty years old,
    - with an RHR of 75 bpm, and
    - a desired intensity of 65 percent.

The Karvonen Formula is as follows:
1. (MHR − RHR) = HRR
2. HRR x Aerobic Intensity + RHR = THR

Explaining the four-step formula:
1. Calculate the maximum heart rate (MHR), which is 220 − age.
2. Deduct the resting heart rate (RHR), and that gives you the heart rate reserve (HRR).
3. Multiply the HRR by the desired aerobic intensity. (It is very important that the intensity selected is between 50–85 percent).
4. Add the RHR.

This gives you the desired training heart rate (THR).

Applying this to our example, the calculation looks like this:
1. **Calculate** the maximum heart rate (220 − 50 = 170)
2. **Deduct** the person's resting heart rate (170 − 75 = 95)
3. **Multiply** by the desired intensity (95 x 0.60 = 61.75)
4. **Add** the person's resting heart rate (**61.75 + 75 = 137**)

The desired training heart rate is 137 beats per minute.

5.2.11

How to Train Safely

The most important things to consider are the following:

- The following suggestions are based on the Maximum Heart Rate (MHR).

- Always consider your age, the length of time you have been training, your fitness level, and the condition of your health.

- As a guideline for beginners in good health, select an aerobics exercise program that uses your maximum heart rate (220 – your age).

- Using the calculation of the maximum heart rate from above, calculate heart rate intensities of 60 percent and 75 percent to determine the lower and upper limits for your aerobic workout.

- If you are over age fifty, or have medical problems:
    - consult your physician before starting your fitness program,
    - or intensifying your fitness program by moving up to the next higher level.

- The primary goals of your aerobic training should be to improve your cardiovascular function and to burn calories.

- In order to continually improve, you must attempt to increase both the intensity and the duration of the aerobic exercise program.

- <u>Once again, for beginners</u>, once you have reached the recommended maximum heart rate of 75 percent, and can sustain that rate for at least 20 minutes, you should attempt to continue at that level for several weeks. Afterward, consult a personal trainer for advice.

- If you are in the intermediate stage as an exerciser, you may select a Training Heart Rate Range in accordance with your fitness level.

- If you are a super athlete, you may train as high as 90 percent of the MHR for your age, however, you should first consult a personal trainer, or your physician, regardless of your age.

- Caution, if you are not a professional athlete, you should <u>never</u> train at or near 90 percent of your MHR.

5.3 Circulatory System Injuries and Conditions

5.3.1

Heart Conditions

- Arrhythmia
- Bradycardia
- Tachycardia
- Aortic Stenosis
- Angina
- Ischemia
- Arteriosclerosis
- Atherosclerosis
- Coronary Artery Disease
- Myocardial Infarction (Heart Attack)
- Myocarditis

Arrhythmia
- Any abnormal rhythm in the way the heart beats.

Bradycardia
- The term used to describe a slow heart rate, one that is less than sixty beats per minute.

Tachycardia
- The term used to describe a rapid heart rate, one that is more than one hundred beats per minute.
- An *electrocardiogram* (a line graph) shows changes in the electrical activity of the heart over time and is made by an instrument called an *electrocardiograph*. The graph can show that there are abnormal conditions, such as blocked arteries, changes in electrolytes (particles with electrical charges), and changes in the way electrical currents pass through the heart tissue. Also called ECG and EKG.

Aortic Stenosis
- This condition is due to the narrowing of the aortic valve opening from the left ventricle of the heart.

Angina
- Pain originating from the heart usually caused by decreased blood flow through the coronary arteries supplying oxygen to the heart. It is also referred to as *angina pectoris*.

Ischemia
- A localized deficiency of blood supply resulting from constriction or obstruction of the arteries.
- This condition results in an insufficient supply of blood to a specific organ or to specific tissues. It is usually caused by atherosclerosis.

Arteriosclerosis
- A thickening and hardening of the artery walls caused by one or more of several diseases.

Atherosclerosis
- A form of arteriosclerosis characterized by the accumulation of calcium, cholesterol, and other fatty materials on the inner walls of the arteries causing them to harden, thicken, and lose elasticity.

Coronary Artery Disease (CAD)
- The specific condition of atherosclerosis when it affects the coronary artery of the heart.

Myocardial Infarction (commonly called a heart attack)
- The death of a section of the heart muscle that occurs when a coronary artery becomes completely blocked. This blockage is usually caused by a blood clot in the coronary artery that has been narrowed by atherosclerosis.

Myocarditis
- A condition that results in inflammation of the heart muscle.
- Occasionally, when an apparently healthy young person has died unexpectedly during participation in a sport, an autopsy reveals the cause of death to be myocarditis.

5.3.2

Blood Conditions

- **Anemia**
- **Cyanosis**
- **Hypercholesterolemia**

Anemia
- A below-normal amount of hemoglobin, which is the oxygen-carrying pigment in the blood.
- Hemoglobin is found inside red blood cells and its purpose is to transport oxygen from the lungs to the tissues of the body.
- The most common type of anemia is due to a deficiency of iron. However, there are many other types of anemia.

Cyanosis
- A bluish discoloration, especially of the skin and mucous membranes, caused by reduced hemoglobin in the blood.

Hypercholesterolemia
- High levels of blood cholesterol.

5.3.3

Understanding Cholesterol

- **Cholesterol** is a soft, waxy substance that belongs to a family of fat compounds called lipids.

- It is manufactured in the body by the liver, and it can also be obtained from any food or drink that comes from animal sources (e.g., meat, poultry, fish, eggs, cheese, butter, etc.).

- Other important characteristics are as follows:

    - Measurements are essential in helping physicians diagnose a person's health.
    - Essential to life.
    - Always present in the blood and in all the cells of the body.
    - Unable to dissolve in the blood.
    - Transported throughout the bloodstream on substances known as lipoproteins.
    - Not found in fruits or vegetables or in any plant.
    - Has many functions, including the building of cell membranes, and the building of brain and nerve tissues.
    - Used to help the body produce steroid hormones, which are needed for body regulation, including the processing of food.
    - Helps the body produce bile acids, which are needed for digestion.
    - Required for other functions of the body's chemistry.

- Cholesterol intake from foods should not exceed 300 milligrams per day.

- Cholesterol is dangerous for the body only when it is present at unhealthy levels.

5.3.4

Cholesterol Terms

- **Lipoproteins**
- **HDL (High-Density Lipoprotein)**
- **LDL (Low-Density Lipoprotein)**
- **Triglycerides**
- **Total Blood Cholesterol**
- **Lipids**

Lipoproteins
- Particles of proteins, cholesterol, and triglycerides that are combined by the liver.
- Their purpose is to <u>transport cholesterol and triglycerides</u> through the blood stream, and therefore throughout the body.

HDL (High-Density Lipoprotein)
- HDL protects the body by transporting cholesterol from cells in the arteries to the liver and other parts of the body for reprocessing or elimination.
- HDLs <u>contain more protein than fat</u> and are referred to as the "good cholesterol" because of their ability to remove cholesterol from the cells in the arteries. This process helps to protect you from having a heart attack or stroke.
- The higher your HDL, the lower your risk. The lower your HDL, the higher your risk.

LDL (Low-Density Lipoprotein)
- LDL transports cholesterol from the liver for use by all the cells of the body.
- LDLs <u>contain more fat than protein</u>.
- LDLs are referred to as the "bad cholesterol" because they also cause build-ups of plaque in the arteries by depositing harmful cholesterol on the artery walls.
- The higher your LDL, the higher your risk. The lower your LDL, the lower your risk.
- Most of the body's cholesterol is LDL cholesterol.

Triglycerides
- The main type of fat consumed in the diet.
- Most of the body's stored fat is in the form of triglycerides.
- Triglycerides are just one type of fat that is transported through the blood to be used by the body's tissues.
- Triglycerides are formed from three fatty acid molecules and one glycerol molecule.
- It is believed that triglycerides may be a risk factor for heart attack or stroke.

Total Blood Cholesterol
- HDL + LDL + 20 percent of a person's triglyceride level.

Lipids
- A group of fatty substances that include cholesterol and triglycerides.
- Lipids are also vital nutrients that are a necessary part of every cell.
- They store energy, supply energy, protect internal organs, and carry fat-soluble vitamins.
- Lipids are also characterized by the fact that they are insoluble in water.

5.3.5

Cholesterol Range References

This chart is a guideline.
Please check with your doctor to be sure that this guideline is appropriate for you.

Definition of mg/dl:
A measurement that means milligrams per deciliter.

Test Name	Reference Range	Units
Total Cholesterol	10–199	mg/dl
HDL Cholesterol	40–125	mg/dl
Triglycerides	10–149	mg/dl
LDL Cholesterol	129 or less	mg/dl
Cholesterol/HDL Ratio	3.4–9.6	RATIO

5.3.6

Dietary Fat and Cholesterol Levels

- Effects of Eating Less Cholesterol
- Effects of Eating Good Cholesterol
- Dietary Cholesterol Requirements
- Cholesterol in Plants and Animals

Effects of Eating Less Cholesterol
- Many people are confused about the effect of dietary fats on cholesterol levels. At first glance, it seems reasonable to think that eating less cholesterol would reduce a person's cholesterol level. Actually, eating less cholesterol has less effect on blood cholesterol levels than eating less saturated fat. However, some studies have found that eating cholesterol increases the risk of heart disease even if it doesn't increase blood cholesterol levels.

Effects of Eating Good Cholesterol
- Another misconception about cholesterol is that people can improve their cholesterol numbers by selecting foods that contain only "good cholesterol." However, this is not possible. When we eat food, our bodies determine whether it will convert the cholesterol to the HDL ("good cholesterol") or the LDL ("bad cholesterol"). We have no say in the matter! In food all cholesterol is the same. In the blood, whether cholesterol is "good" or "bad" depends on the type of lipoprotein that's carrying it.

Dietary Cholesterol Requirements
- People don't need to consume any dietary cholesterol because the body can make enough cholesterol for all of its needs. The typical American diet contains substantial amounts of cholesterol, however, which is found in foods such as egg yolks, liver, meat, some shellfish, and whole-milk dairy products.

Cholesterol in Plants and Animals
- The **only** foods that contain cholesterol are foods of animal origin.
- <u>Plant foods do not contain cholesterol.</u>

5.3.7

Blood Vessel Conditions

- **Aneurysm**
- **Stroke (Cerebrovascular Accident)**
  - **Cerebral Thrombosis**
  - **Cerebral Embolism**
  - **Cerebral Hemorrhage**
- **Stroke Symptoms**
- **Range of Stroke Damage**
- **Risk Factors For Stroke**

Aneurysm
- A bubble in a blood vessel that creates a weak spot in the wall of the vessel. The condition can be fatal if it ruptures.
- It is possible to have a genetic predisposition to develop aneurysms.

Stroke
- Each of these three types of strokes is referred to as a *cerebrovascular accident* (CVA).

  - **Cerebral Thrombosis**: An impaired blood supply to the brain caused by a blood clot.

  - **Cerebral Embolism**: A ruptured blood vessel in the brain that had been weakened by a bubble in that vessel.

  - **Cerebral Hemorrhage**: A ruptured blood vessel in the brain.

Stroke Symptoms
- Headache
- Dizziness
- Confusion
- Visual disturbance
- Slurred speech
- Loss of speech
- Difficulty swallowing

Range of Stroke Damage
- Damage from a stroke ranges from unnoticeable, to mild or severe loss of bodily function (e.g., slurred speech, weakness or paralysis on one side of the body), to death.
- Very often immediate emergency care in a hospital cannot only save the patient's life, but it can also reduce the degree of damage.
- It is of utmost importance that the patient be brought to a hospital within thirty minutes of experiencing symptoms to minimize the consequences.

Risk Factors For Stroke
- Age
- High blood pressure
- Atherosclerosis
- Heart disease
- Diabetes mellitus
- Smoking
- Use of estrogens

CHAPTER 6

The Respiratory System

6.1 Anatomy of the Respiratory System ·····························299
    6.1.1   Respiratory System ··301
    6.1.2   Airway Components······································304
    6.1.3   Pulmonary Blood Vessels ·······························310
    6.1.4   Muscles Used for Breathing ····························311

6.2 Respiratory System Injuries and Conditions ····················315
    6.2.1   Respiratory Conditions ··································317
    6.2.2   Breathing Abnormalities ································319

6.1 Anatomy of the Respiratory System

6.1.1

Respiratory System

- **Airways**
- **Lungs**
- **Linked Blood Vessels**

Introduction to the Respiratory System:

- The **respiratory system** is made up of organs and tissues that help you breathe.

- The main parts of this system are the **airways, the lungs, linked blood vessels**, and the muscles that enable breathing.

- When the respiratory system is mentioned, people generally think of breathing, but breathing is only one of the activities of the respiratory system.

- The body cells need a continuous supply of oxygen for the metabolic processes that are necessary to maintain life.

- The respiratory system works with the circulatory system to provide this oxygen and to remove the waste products of metabolism.

- It also helps to regulate pH of the blood.

- Respiration is the sequence of events that results in the exchange of oxygen and carbon dioxide between the atmosphere and the body cells.

- Every 3 to 5 seconds, nerve impulses stimulate the breathing process, or ventilation, which moves air through a series of passages into and out of the lungs.

- After this, there is an exchange of gases between the lungs and the blood. <u>This is called external respiration</u>.

- The blood transports the gases to and from the tissue cells.

- The exchange of gases between the blood and tissue cells is <u>internal respiration</u>.

- Finally, the cells utilize the oxygen for their specific activities: <u>this is called cellular metabolism, or cellular respiration</u>.

- Together, these activities constitute respiration.

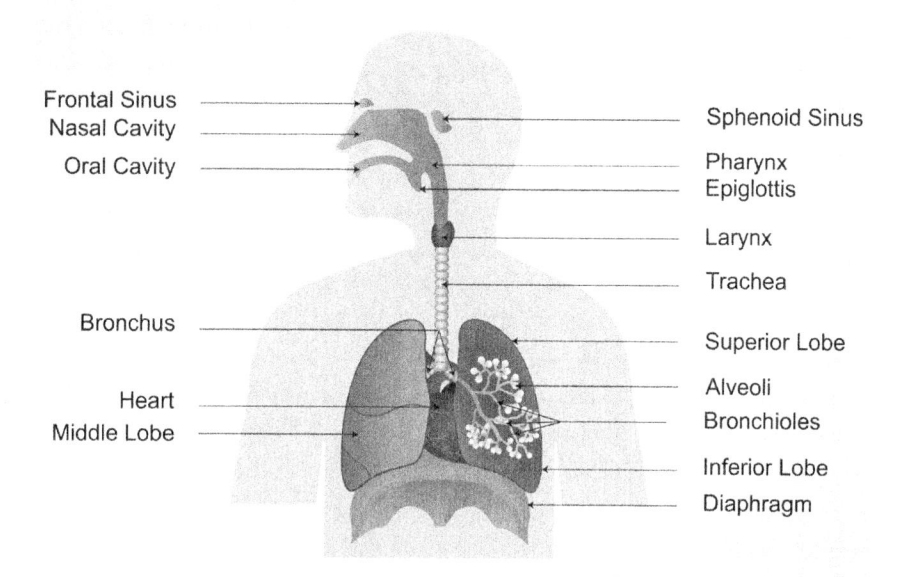

Frontal Sinus
Nasal Cavity
Oral Cavity

Sphenoid Sinus
Pharynx
Epiglottis
Larynx
Trachea

Bronchus

Superior Lobe
Alveoli
Bronchioles
Inferior Lobe
Diaphragm

Heart
Middle Lobe

6.1.2

Airway Components

The Upper Respiratory Tract

- Airways
- Frontal Sinus
- Sphenoid Sinus
- Nose and Mouth
- Pharynx (Throat)
- Larynx (Voice Box)
- Epiglottis
- Cilia

The Lower Respiratory Tract

- Trachea (Windpipe)
- Bronchus (plural is Bronchi)
- Bronchi
- Bronchioles
- Alveolar Ducts
- Alveoli
- Lobes
- Fissures
- Pleura
- Bronchial Tree
- Lungs

The Upper Respiratory Tract:

Airways
- Within the respiratory system are pipes that carry oxygen-rich air to the lungs. They also carry carbon dioxide, a waste gas, out of the lungs.

Frontal Sinus
- A type of paranasal sinus (a hollow space in the bones around the nose).
- There are two, large frontal sinuses in the frontal bone, which forms the lower part of the forehead and reaches over the eye sockets and eyebrows.
- The frontal sinuses are lined with cells that make mucus to keep the nose from drying out.

Sphenoid Sinus
- A type of paranasal sinus (a hollow space in the bones around the nose).
- There are two large sphenoid sinuses in the sphenoid bone, which is behind the nose between the eyes.
- The sphenoid sinuses are lined with cells that make mucus to keep the nose from drying out.

Nose and Mouth
- Air first enters your body through your nose or mouth, which wet and warm the air (because cold, dry air can irritate your lungs).

Pharynx (Throat)
- The hollow tube inside the neck that starts behind the nose and ends at the top of the *trachea* (windpipe) and *esophagus* (the tube that goes to the stomach).
- The pharynx is about five inches long, depending on body size.

Larynx (Voice Box) and Trachea (Windpipe)
- From the pharynx, air then travels through your *larynx* (or voice box) and down your *trachea* (windpipe).

Epiglottis (Adam's Apple)
- A thin flap of tissue called the *epiglottis* covers your windpipe when you swallow. This prevents food and drink from entering the air passages that lead to your lungs.

Cilia
- Except for the mouth and some parts of the nose, all the airways have special hairs called *cilia* that are coated with sticky mucus.
- The cilia trap germs and other foreign particles that enter your airways when you breathe in air. These fine hairs then sweep the particles up to the nose or mouth.
- From there, they're swallowed, coughed, or sneezed out of the body.
- Nose hairs and mouth saliva also trap particles and germs.

The Lower Respiratory Tract:

Trachea
- The trachea, commonly called the windpipe, is the main airway to the lungs. It divides into the right and left bronchi at the level of the fifth thoracic vertebra, channeling air to the right or left lung.

Bronchus
- The *trachea* splits into two *bronchus* (a left and a right).

Bronchi (Plural of Bronchus)
- Each main bronchus subdivides into smaller airway passages referred to as *bronchi*.

Bronchioles
- Within the lungs, the bronchi branch into thousands of smaller, thinner tubes called bronchioles.

Alveolar Ducts
- As the *bronchioles* proceed further into the lungs, they become thinner, and develop into *alveolar ducts*.

Alveoli
- The alveolar ducts end in tiny round **air sacs** that contain clusters of cup shaped **alveoli.**
- Each of these **air sacs** is covered in a mesh of tiny blood vessels called capillaries.
- The alveoli are the center of respiratory function of the lungs.
- The pulmonary artery and its branches deliver blood rich in carbon dioxide (and lacking in oxygen) to the capillaries that surround the air sacs.
- Inside the air sacs, carbon dioxide moves from the blood into the air.
- At the same time, oxygen moves from the air into the blood in the capillaries.
- The oxygen-rich blood then travels to the heart through the pulmonary vein and its branches.
- The heart pumps the oxygen-rich blood out to the body.

Lobes
- The lungs consist of five lobes.
- Each lung receives air from its own bronchus.
- The right lung has three lobes and the left has two.
- The left lung has a superior and inferior lobe.
- The right lung has superior, middle, and inferior lobes.
- Each lobe is separated from the other by *fissures* (partitions) to protect against disease or mechanical injury.
    - Though some people need to have a diseased lung lobe removed, they can still breathe well using the rest of their lung lobes.

Fissures
- The thin walls of tissue that separate the different lobes.

Pleura
- A double layered membrane that encloses each lung.
- It also lines the chest cavity.
- The small space between the layers of the pleura is called the *pleural cavity*.
- It contains a thin film of fluid that is produced by the pleura.
- The fluid acts as a lubricant to reduce friction as the two layers slide against each other, and it helps to hold the two layers together as the lungs expand during inhalation, and contract during exhalation.
- The pleura also provides protection against disease.

Bronchial Tree
- The combination of:
- the trachea
- the two primary bronchi
- the alveolar ducts
- the alveolar sacs
- the alveoli, located at the at the end of the bronchial tree.
- The entire bronchial tree has a covering of veins and arteries that go into and out of the lungs.

Lungs
- The lungs and linked blood vessels deliver oxygen to, and remove carbon dioxide from your body.
- They are the major organs of the respiratory system, and are divided into two sections called lobes:
    1. The right lung is slightly larger than the left lung, and has three lobes.
    2. The left lung has two lobes.
- The lungs are soft and spongy because they are mostly air spaces surrounded by the alveolar cells and elastic connective tissue.
- They are <u>separated from each other</u> by the *mediastinum* (the area that contains the heart, trachea, esophagus, and many lymph nodes).
- The trachea, which begins at the edge of the larynx, divides into two bronchi, and continues into the lungs.
- The bronchi divide into smaller bronchioles, which branch out in the lungs forming passageways for air.
- The terminal parts of the bronchi are the alveoli.
- The alveoli are the functional units of the lungs and they form the site of <u>gaseous exchange</u> (delivering oxygen to, and removing carbon dioxide from your body).

6.1.3

Pulmonary Blood Vessels

- **Pulmonary Artery**
- **Pulmonary Vein**

Pulmonary Artery
- The pulmonary artery and its branches deliver blood rich in carbon dioxide (and lacking in oxygen) to the capillaries that surround the alveoli.
- Inside the alveoli, carbon dioxide moves from the blood into the air. At the same time, oxygen moves from the air into the blood in the capillaries.

Pulmonary Vein
- The oxygen-rich blood then travels to the heart through the pulmonary vein and its branches. The heart pumps the oxygen-rich blood out to the body.

6.1.4

Muscles Used for Breathing

- **Diaphragm**
- **Intercostal Muscles**
- **Abdominal Muscles**
- **Upon Inhalation**
- **Upon Exhalation**

- Muscles near the lungs help expand and contract the lungs to allow breathing.
- Muscles in your neck and collarbone area help you breathe in when other muscles involved in breathing don't work well, or when lung disease impairs your breathing.

Diaphragm
- A dome-shaped muscle located below your lungs that separates the chest cavity from the abdominal cavity.
- The diaphragm is the main muscle used for breathing.

Intercostal Muscles
- Located between your ribs, they also play a major role in helping you breathe.

Abdominal Muscles
- Beneath your diaphragm, they help you breathe out when you're breathing fast (for example, during physical activity).

Upon Inhalation
- When you breathe in, or inhale, your diaphragm contracts (tightens) and moves downward. This increases the space in your chest cavity into which your lungs expand.
- The intercostal muscles between your ribs also help enlarge the chest cavity. They contract to pull your rib cage both upward and outward when you inhale.
- As your lungs expand, air is sucked in through your nose or mouth. The air travels down your windpipe and into your lungs.
- After passing through your bronchial tubes, the air finally reaches and enters the alveoli (air sacs).
- Through the very thin walls of the alveoli, oxygen from the air passes to the surrounding capillaries (blood vessels). A red blood cell protein called *hemoglobin* helps move oxygen from the air sacs to the blood.
- At the same time, carbon dioxide moves from the capillaries into the air sacs. The gas has traveled in the bloodstream from the right side of the heart through the pulmonary artery.
- Oxygen-rich blood from the lungs is carried through a network of capillaries to the pulmonary vein. This vein delivers the oxygen-rich blood to the left side of the heart.
- The left side of the heart pumps the blood to the rest of the body. There, the oxygen in the blood moves from blood vessels into surrounding tissues.

Upon Exhalation
- When you breathe out, or exhale, your diaphragm relaxes and moves upward into the chest cavity.
- The intercostal muscles between the ribs also relax to reduce the space in the chest cavity.
- As the space in the chest cavity gets smaller, air rich in carbon dioxide is forced out of your lungs and windpipe, and then out of your nose or mouth.
- Breathing out requires no effort from your body unless you have a lung disease or are doing physical activity.
- When you're physically active, your abdominal muscles contract and push your diaphragm against your lungs even more than usual. This rapidly pushes air out of your lungs.

6.2 Respiratory System Injuries and Conditions

6.2.1

Respiratory Conditions

- **Dyspnea**
- **Suffocation**
- **Bronchitis**
- **Asthma (Bronchial Asthma)**
- **Exercise-Induced Asthma**
- **Cyanosis**
- **Chronic Obstructive Pulmonary Disease**
- **Emphysema**

Dyspnea
- Struggling for air, difficulty breathing, labored breathing.

Suffocation
- A lack of air going into the lungs due to blockage of the air passage.

Bronchitis
- Acute or chronic inflammation of the bronchial tubes, which are the airways that lead to the alveoli in the lungs.
- Results in reduced airflow, mucus build-up, and persistent coughing.

Asthma (Bronchial Asthma)
- Episodes of breathing difficulty and wheezing while breathing out.
- The condition is more accurately referred to as *bronchial asthma* because it differentiates the condition from the wheezing that is associated with heart failure.
- When the wheezing is associated with heart failure, it is more accurately referred to as *cardiac asthma*.

Exercise-Induced Asthma
- For the asthma sufferer, exercise may trigger an asthma attack due to the body's increased demand for oxygen.

Cyanosis
- In cases where an asthma attack is very severe, the individual may suffer from a very low amount of oxygen in the blood, which causes a blue-purple discoloration of the face, especially the lips. This discoloration is referred to as *cyanosis*.
- Additionally, the individual may also suffer from pale and clammy skin.

Chronic Obstructive Pulmonary Disease (COPD)
- Asthma, bronchitis, and emphysema are examples of chronic obstruction of airflow.

Emphysema
- A serious chronic disease of the lungs in which there is damage to, or loss of, the air sacs (alveoli), which results in a shortness of breath.
- In more severe cases, this condition can lead to respiratory failure or heart failure, which can lead to death.

6.2.2

Breathing Abnormalities

- **Valsalva Maneuver**
- **Aerophagia**
- **Hyperventilation**

Valsalva Maneuver
- A condition caused by holding one's breath while straining during the performance of an exercise.
- It is a phenomenon that increases pressure within the chest region and also raises blood pressure.
- It is especially dangerous for people with high blood pressure.
- Always exhale through the mouth during exertion.

Aerophagia
- Excessive swallowing of air.

Hyperventilation
- Abnormally rapid breathing usually resulting from an anxiety or panic attack.
- Other causes of hyperventilation can occur from diabetes mellitus, pulmonary edema, emphysema, or renal failure.
- Hyperventilation results in an abnormal loss of carbon dioxide in the blood and may also cause *alkalosis*, which is an increase in the alkalinity level in the blood. The typical symptoms are dizziness, feeling faint, a numbness or tingling in the extremities, and feeling that breathing is difficult.
- The alkalosis associated with hyperventilation worsens the existing condition of anxiety to such a level that the individual has a sense of impending doom.
- To counter the effects of hyperventilation, it is recommended that an individual breathe into a paper bag so as to increase the level of carbon dioxide in the blood and also to prevent the risk of alkalosis.

CHAPTER 7

The Nervous System

7.1 Anatomy of the Nervous System ·····323
- 7.1.1 Nervous System Divisions ·····325
- 7.1.2 Subdivisions of the Central Nervous System ·····327
- 7.1.3 Subdivisions of the Peripheral Nervous System ·····328
- 7.1.4 Brain Anatomy ·····330
- 7.1.5 Left and Right Brain Functions ·····332
- 7.1.6 Structure of a Typical Neuron ·····333
- 7.1.7 Brain Wave and Electrical Activity Testing ·····336
- 7.1.8 Anatomy of the Spinal Cord ·····337
- 7.1.9 Eyes and Nervous System ·····342
- 7.1.10 Components of Eye Anatomy ·····343
- 7.1.11 Eye Function ·····349

7.2 Nervous System Injuries and Conditions ·····351
- 7.2.1 Seizures (Convulsions) ·····353
- 7.2.2 Health Conditions of the Nervous System ·····355
- 7.2.3 Arthritis Types That May Affect the Spine ·····358
- 7.2.4 Acquired Causes of Spinal Conditions ·····359
- 7.2.5 Eye Conditions ·····362
- 7.2.6 Eye Tests ·····365
- 7.2.7 Eye Surgery and Treatments ·····367

7.1 Anatomy of the Nervous System

7.1.1

Nervous System Divisions

- **Central Nervous System**
- **Peripheral Nervous System**

Nervous System

- An organized network of nerve tissue in the body.
- It includes the central nervous system, the peripheral nervous system, and other nerve tissue.
- Acting together, these divisions transmit signals between different parts of the body to coordinate the body's voluntary and involuntary actions.
- When a part of the nervous system is not functioning properly, which is usually caused by illness, injury, age, genetics, or other reasons, a person may experience difficulty with speaking, learning, swallowing, breathing, moving, memory, senses, mood, or other physical or psychological functions.

Central Nervous System

- Includes the brain and the spinal cord.

Peripheral Nervous System
- Consists of <u>nerves and neurons</u> that are located outside of the brain and spinal cord.
- Connects the central nervous system to the limbs and organs, and relays messages back and forth from the brain and the extremities.

See section 7.1.6 for details about additional nerve tissue.

7.1.2

Subdivisions of the Central Nervous System

- **Brain**
- **Spinal Cord**

Brain
- The body's main control center, the brain is the <u>major organ of the central nervous system</u> and is located inside the skull.
- The brain controls all the functions of the body, such as speaking, learning, behavior, swallowing, breathing, moving, memory, abstract thought, language usage, senses, mood, and much more.

Spinal Cord
- A soft bundle of nerves that are attached to the base of the brain and go down to the lower back through the spinal canal.
- The spinal canal is protected by the bones of the spine, which are known as vertebrae.
- Signals between the brain and the nerve roots travel up and down the spinal cord to enable the brain and body to communicate.
- The vertebrae have disks that provide cushioning and flexibility to the spine and spinal cord.

7.1.3

Subdivisions of the Peripheral Nervous System

- **Autonomic Nervous System**
- **Sympathetic Nervous System**
- **Parasympathetic Nervous System**

Autonomic Nervous System
- Also known as the *visceral nervous system* or *involuntary nervous system*.
- A division of the peripheral nervous system that influences the function of internal organs.
- Its functions are primarily unconscious, yet some do work along with the conscious mind.
- The unconscious autonomic nervous system controls such functions as heart rate, digestion, respiration rate, salivation, perspiration, diameter of the pupils, discharge of urine, sexual arousal, and reflex actions such as coughing, sneezing, swallowing, and vomiting.
- Breathing is an example whereby the conscious and the unconscious autonomic nervous system may work together.
- The autonomic nervous system has two divisions:

Sympathetic Nervous System
- It is responsible for stimulating activities such as causing the body to become active and responsive, especially as it relates to the *fight or flight* response.

Parasympathetic Nervous System
- It is responsible for rest activities and controls the bodies rest and digest or *feed and breed* response.
- This response is activated when the body is at rest, especially after eating, digestion, urination, and defecation.

7.1.4

Brain Anatomy

- **Corpus Callosum**
- **Cerebrum**
- **Cerebellum**
- **Medulla**
- **Brain Weight and Energy Requirements**

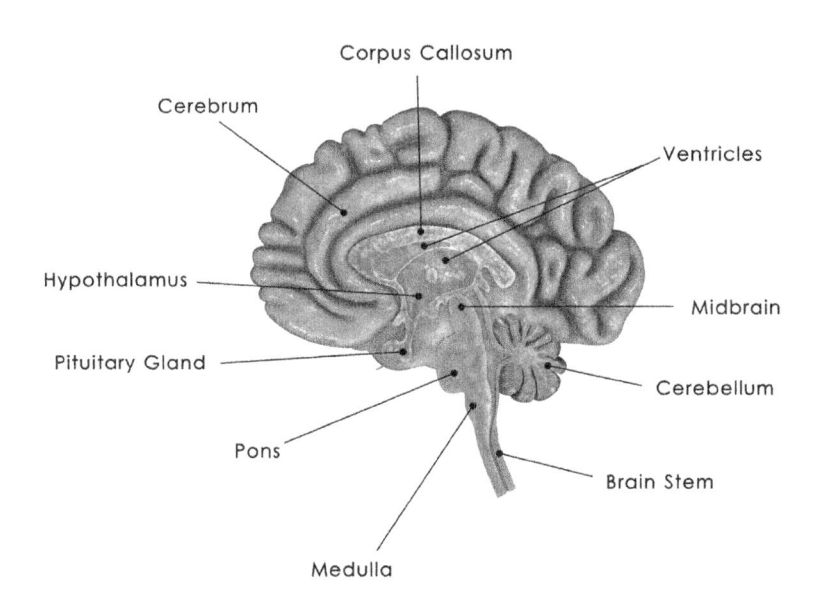

Corpus Callosum
- A large bundle of nerve fibers that connect the left and right cerebral hemispheres of the brain.

Cerebrum
- The forward part of the brain, and also the largest part, that is the central location for memory, thought, and reason, as well as the central location for hearing and sight.

Cerebellum
- Located below the cerebrum, the cerebellum is responsible for controlling muscular coordination, equilibrium, and balance.

Medulla
- The part of the brain that is the <u>enlarged upper end of the spinal cord</u>. It is responsible for controlling breathing, circulation, sneezing, swallowing, and other involuntary activities.

Brain Weight and Energy Requirements
- The energy requirements of the brain are very high.
- The adult brain weighs approximately 3.3 pounds, which is about 2.7 percent of our total body weight.
- About 20 percent of the heart's output (at rest) is necessary to keep the brain functioning.
- The brain requires more oxygen for its tissue cells than any other tissue cells of the body. In fact, the oxygen needs are so great that if there is no circulation to the brain for only ten seconds, a person will become unconscious.

7.1.5

Left and Right Brain Functions

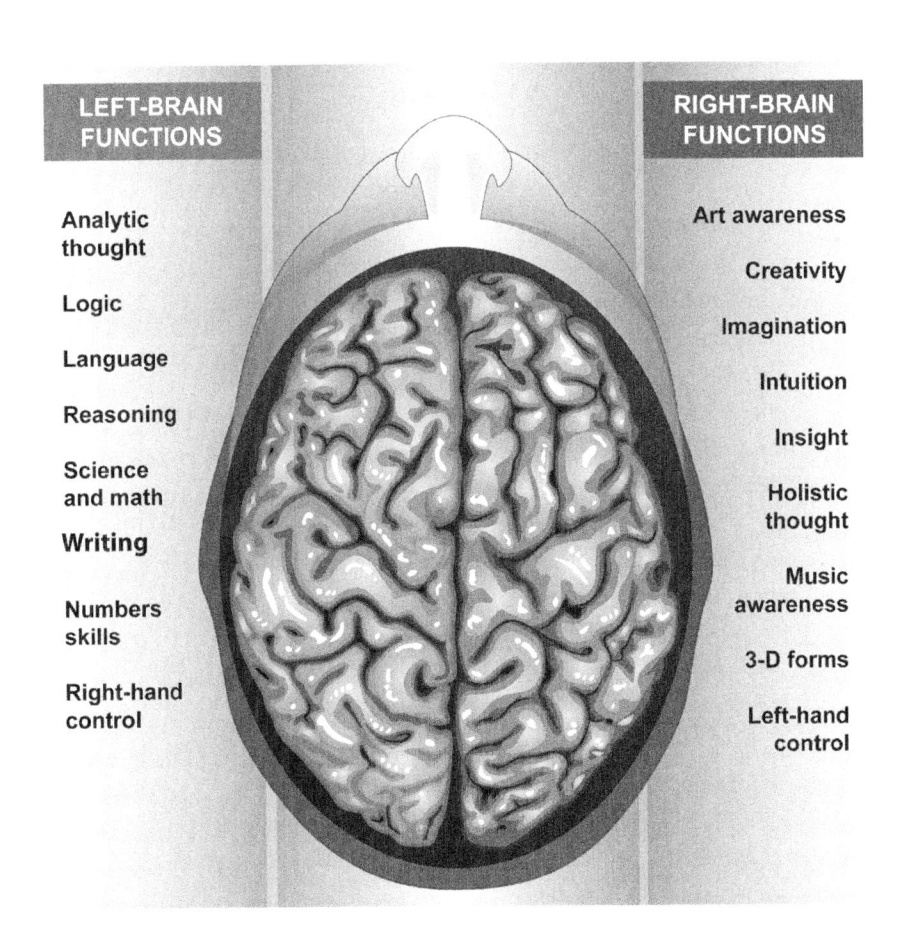

LEFT-BRAIN FUNCTIONS

Analytic thought

Logic

Language

Reasoning

Science and math

Writing

Numbers skills

Right-hand control

RIGHT-BRAIN FUNCTIONS

Art awareness

Creativity

Imagination

Intuition

Insight

Holistic thought

Music awareness

3-D forms

Left-hand control

7.1.6

Structure of a Typical Neuron

- **Nerve Tissue**
- **Neuroglia**
- **Neurons**
- **Soma**
- **Dendrites**
- **Axon**
- **Myelin**
- **Nodes of Ranvier**
- **Oligodendrocytes**
- **Schwann Cells**

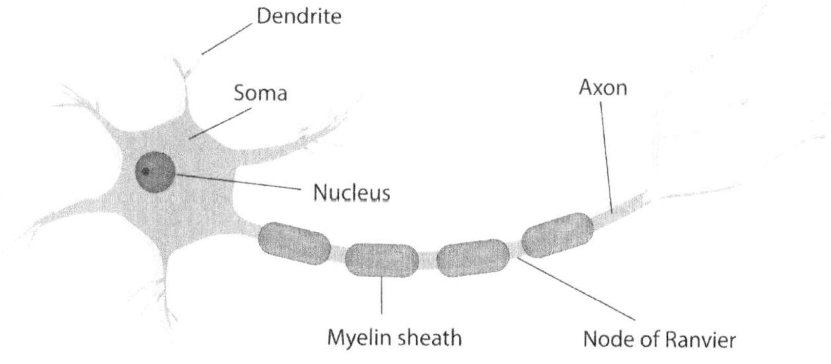
Dendrite
Soma
Axon
Nucleus
Myelin sheath
Node of Ranvier

Nerve Tissue

- Although the nervous system is very complex, there are only two main types of cells in nerve tissue:
    1. The actual nerve cell is the *neuron*. It is the "conducting" cell that transmits impulses and the structural unit of the nervous system.
    2. The other type of cell is *neuroglia, or glial* cell.

Neuroglia
- The word *neuroglia* means "nerve glue." These cells are nonconductive and provide a support system for the neurons.
- They are a special type of connective tissue for the nervous system.

Neurons
- Neurons, or nerve cells, carry out the functions of the nervous system by conducting nerve impulses.
- They are highly specialized and *amitotic*.
- Amitotic means that if a neuron is destroyed, it <u>cannot be replaced</u> because neurons do not go through *mitosis* (the part of the cell cycle in which chromosomes in a nucleus are separated into two identical sets of chromosomes, and each set ends up in its own nucleus.)
  - Each neuron has three basic parts:
    1. Soma
    2. One or more dendrites
    3. A single axon

Soma
- The cell body.

Dendrites
- The branched projections of a neuron that act to propagate the electrochemical stimulation received from other neural cells to the cell body, or *soma*, of the neuron, from which the dendrites project.

Axon
- A long, slender projection of a nerve cell, or neuron, that typically conducts electrical impulses away from the neuron's cell body.
- The function of the axon is to transmit information to different neurons, muscles, and glands.

Myelin
- There are two types of axons occurring in the peripheral nervous system and the central nervous system: unmyelinated and myelinated axons.
- Myelin is a layer of a fatty insulating substance, which is formed by two types of glial cells: *Schwann cells* ensheathing peripheral neurons and *oligodendrocytes* insulating those of the central nervous system.

Nodes of Ranvier
- Gaps in the myelin sheath at evenly spaced intervals along myelinated nerve fibers.
- Myelination enables an especially rapid mode of electrical impulse propagation called *saltatory conduction*.
- Demyelination of axons causes the multitude of neurological symptoms found in the disease *multiple sclerosis*.

Oligodendrocytes
- A type of neuroglia, the main functions of which are to provide support and insulation to axons in the central nervous system of some vertebrates. Oligodendrocytes do this by creating the myelin sheath.
- Equivalent to the function performed by Schwann cells in the peripheral nervous system.

Schwann Cells
- They are the principal glia of the peripheral nervous system
- Glial cells function to support neurons.

7.1.7

Brain Wave and Electrical Activity Testing

Electroencephalogram (EEG)
- An EEG test is performed to detect abnormal brain waves. It also detects the electrical activity of the brain.
- This test requires the use of electrodes that are pasted onto the scalp. These electrodes are small metal discs with thin wires.
- EEG results are printed out as a graph on a computer, as well as amplified and recorded for evaluation by a doctor.

7.1.8

Anatomy of the Spinal Cord

- Spine
- Vertebral Column
- Intervertebral Disks
- Facet Joints
- Ligaments
- Pedicles
- Synovium
- Vertebral Arch
- Intervertebral Foramen (Neural Foramen)
- Lamina
- Ligamentum Flavum
- Cauda Equina

Spinal Cord
- A major part of the central nervous system that extends from the base of the brain down to the lower back and is encased by the vertebral column.
- Consists of nerve cells and bundles of nerves that are covered by three thin layers of protective tissue called membranes.
- The cord connects the brain to all parts of the body via thirty-one pairs of nerves that branch out from the cord and leave the spine between vertebrae (back bones).

Spine
- All of the bones, muscles, tendons, and other tissues that reach from the base of the skull to the tailbone.
- The spine encloses the spinal cord and the fluid surrounding the spinal cord.
- Also called the *backbone, spinal column,* or *vertebral column.*

Vertebral Column
- Protects the spinal cord from injury.
- Encloses the spinal cord and the fluid surrounding it.
- See a list of bones of the vertebral column in section 2.1.6.

Intervertebral Disks
- The pads of cartilage that are filled with a gel-like substance that lie between vertebrae and act as shock absorbers.

SPEED LEARNING FOR ANATOMY

Normal Disc & Disc Conditions

Disc (correct spelling)
- Spelling with a "c" (disc) is proper in anatomy, though it is often spelled with a "k" (disk). Both are acceptable.
- They can be used interchangeably, and both versions are used in this book.

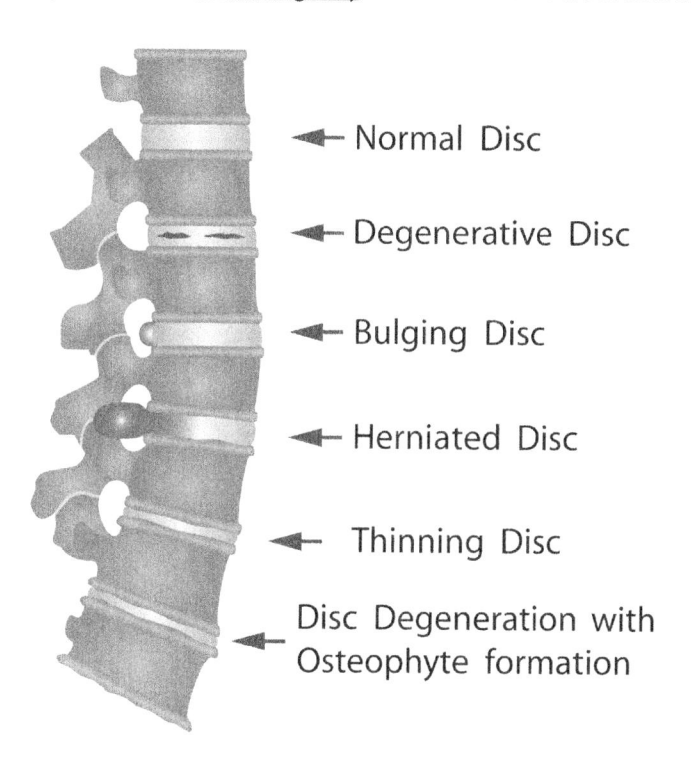

← Normal Disc

← Degenerative Disc

← Bulging Disc

← Herniated Disc

← Thinning Disc

← Disc Degeneration with Osteophyte formation

Facet Joints
- Connect the vertebrae to each other and permit backward motion.

Ligaments
- The elastic bands of tissue that support the spine by preventing the vertebrae from slipping out of line as the spine moves.

Pedicles
- These are the narrow stem-like structures on the vertebrae that form the walls of the front part of the vertebral arch.

Synovium
- This is a thin membrane that produces fluid to lubricate the facet joints and allow them to move easily.

Vertebral Arch
- A circle of bone around the spinal canal through which the spinal cord passes.
- Composed of a floor at the back of the vertebra, walls (the pedicles), and a ceiling where two laminae join.

Intervertebral Foramen (or Neural Foramen)
- An opening between the vertebrae through which nerves leave the spine and extend to other parts of the body.

Lamina
- A part of the vertebra at the back portion of the vertebral arch that forms the roof of the canal through which the spinal cord and nerve roots pass.

Ligamentum Flavum
- A large ligament that is often involved in spinal stenosis. It runs as a continuous band from lamina to lamina in the spine.

Cauda Equina
- A sack of nerve roots that continues from the lumbar region, where the spinal cord ends, and continues down to provide neurologic function to the lower part of the body.
- It resembles a horse's tail.

7.1.9

Eyes and Nervous System

- The eyes are a component of the **central nervous system**.

- The images seen through the eyes are transmitted by the nervous system to the brain.

- The eye is designed to focus an image onto the *retina*, which is located at the back of the eye, and the nerve that carries the image from the *retina* to the brain is the *optic nerve*.

7.1.10

Components of Eye Anatomy

- Cornea
- Iris
- Lens
- Pupil
- Retina
- Macula
- Optic Nerve
- Anterior Chamber
- Aqueous Fluid (Aqueous Humor)
- Blind Spot
- Central Retinal Artery
- Central Retinal Vein
- Choroid
- Ciliary Muscles
- Ciliary Processes
- Cones (Cone Cells)
- Conjunctiva
- Drusen
- Fovea
- Fundus
- Lacrimal Gland
- Optic Cup
- Optic Disc (Optic Nerve Head)
- Retinal Pigment Epithelium
- Rods (Rod Cells)
- Schlemm's Canal
- Sclera
- Trabecular Meshwork
- Uvea (Uveal Tract)
- Posterior Chamber
- Vitreous Humor
- Zonules
- Stroma
- Endothelium
- Epithelium

Eye Anatomy

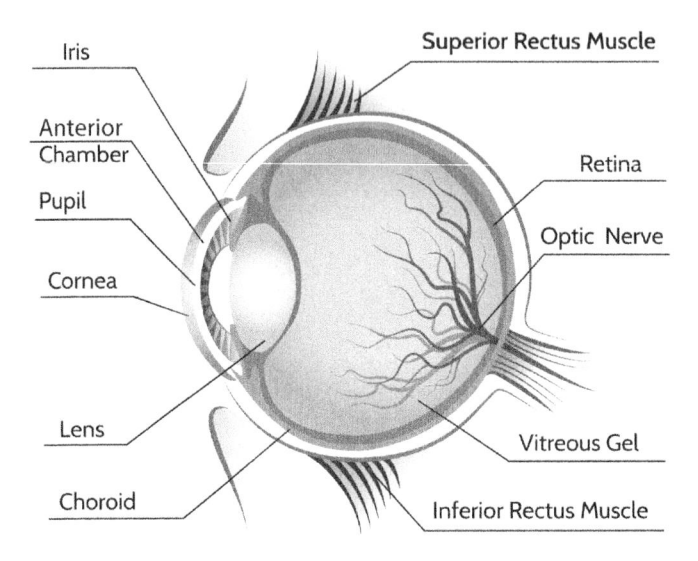

Cornea
- The outer, transparent, dome-like structure that covers the iris, pupil, and anterior chamber. It is part of the eye's focusing system.

Iris
- The colored ring of tissue suspended behind the cornea and immediately in front of the lens. It regulates the amount of light entering the eye by adjusting the size of the pupil.

Lens
- The transparent, double convex structure suspended between the *aqueous humor* and *vitreous humor*. It helps to focus light on the retina.

Pupil
- The adjustable opening at the center of the iris that allows varying amounts of light to enter the eye.

Retina
- The light-sensitive layer of tissue that lines the back of the eyeball.
- It sends visual messages through the optic nerve to the brain

Macula
- The small, sensitive area of the central retina that provides vision for fine work and reading.

Optic Nerve
- The bundle of over one million nerve fibers that carry visual messages from the retina to the brain.

Anterior Chamber
- The space in front of the iris and behind the cornea.

Aqueous Fluid (Aqueous Humor)
- The clear, watery fluid that flows between and nourishes the lens and the cornea. It is secreted by the ciliary processes.

Blind Spot
- A small area of the retina where the optic nerve enters the eye. It occurs normally in all eyes.

Central Retinal Artery
- The blood vessel that carries blood into eye and supplies nutrition to the retina.

Central Retinal Vein
- The blood vessel that carries blood from the retina.

Choroid
- The layer filled with blood vessels that nourish the retina. It is part of the uvea.

Ciliary Muscles
- The muscles that relax the zonules to enable the lens to change shape for focusing.

Ciliary Processes
- The extensions or projections of the ciliary body that secrete aqueous humor.

Cones (Cone Cells)
- One type of specialized light-sensitive cells (photoreceptors) in the retina that provide sharp central vision and color vision. *See also Rods.*

Conjunctiva
- The thin, moist tissue (membrane) that lines the inner surfaces of the eyelids and the outer surface of the sclera.

Drusen
- Tiny yellow or white deposits in the retina or optic nerve head.

Fovea
- The central part of the macula that provides the sharpest vision.

Fundus
- The interior lining of the eyeball, including the retina, optic disc, and macula. It is the portion of the inner eye that can be seen during an eye examination by looking through the pupil.

Lacrimal Gland
- The small almond-shaped structure that produces tears and is located just above the outer corner of the eye.

Optic Cup
- The white, cup-like area in the center of the optic disc.

Optic Disc (Optic Nerve Head)
- The circular area (disc) where the optic nerve connects to the retina.

Retinal Pigment Epithelium (RPE)
- The pigment cell layer that nourishes the retinal cells. It is located just outside the retina and attached to the choroid.

Rods (Rod Cells)
- One type of specialized light-sensitive cells (photoreceptors) in the retina that provide side vision and the ability to see objects in dim light (night vision).

Schlemm's Canal
- The passageway for the aqueous fluid to leave the eye.

Sclera
- The tough, white, outer layer (coat) of the eyeball. Along with the cornea, it protects the entire eyeball.

Trabecular Meshwork
- The spongy, mesh-like tissue near the front of the eye that allows the aqueous fluid (humor) to flow to Schlemm's canal then out of the eye through ocular veins.

Uvea (Uveal Tract)
- The middle coat of the eyeball, consisting of the choroid in the back of the eye and the ciliary body and iris in the front of the eye.

Posterior Chamber
- The space between the back of the iris and the front face of the vitreous. It is filled with aqueous fluid.

Vitreous Humor
- The transparent, colorless mass of gel that lies behind the lens and in front of the retina and fills the center of the eyeball.

Zonules
- The fibers that hold the lens suspended in position and enable it to change shape during accommodation.

Stroma
- The middle, thickest layer of tissue in the cornea.

Endothelium
- The inner layer of cells on the inside surface of the cornea.

Epithelium
- The outermost layer of cells of the cornea and the eye's first defense against infection.

7.1.11

Eye Function

- Accommodation
- Binocular Vision
- Contrast Sensitivity
- Intraocular Pressure (IOP)
- Peripheral Vision
- Visual Acuity
- Visual Field
- Acuity
- Refractive Power

Accommodation
- The ability of the eye to change its focus from distant to near objects. This process is achieved by the lens changing its shape.

Binocular Vision
- The blending of the separate images seen by each eye into a single image. It allows images to be seen with depth.

Contrast Sensitivity
- The ability to perceive differences between an object and its background.

Intraocular Pressure (IOP)
- Pressure of the fluid inside the eye.
- Normal IOP varies among individuals.

Peripheral Vision
- The ability to see objects and movement outside of the direct line of vision. Also called *side vision.*

Visual Acuity
- The ability to distinguish details and shapes of objects. It is also called *central vision.*

Visual Field
- The entire area that can be seen when the eye is forward, including peripheral vision.

Acuity
- The clearness or sharpness of vision.

Refractive Power
- The ability of the eye to bend light as light passes through it.

7.2 Nervous System Injuries and Conditions

7.2.1

Seizures (Convulsions)

- **Epilepsy**
- **Grand Mal Seizure**
- **Aura**
- **Tonic Phase**
- **Clonic Phase**
- **Postictal Phase**

Seizures (Convulsions)
- The sudden occurrence of <u>abnormal electrical activity in the brain</u>.
- A seizure can affect sensation, behavior, movement, or consciousness.
- In a mild seizure, the victim may experience tingling, twitching, hallucinations, familiarity (déjà vu), or fear.
- In a more severe seizure, the victim may experience unconsciousness.
- Seizures can result from many causes that affect brain function, including:
    - Neurological conditions
    - Medical conditions such as an infection, metabolic abnormalities, alcohol withdrawal, poison, and high fever
    - Decreased oxygen supply to the brain
    - Head injuries
    - Brain irritation
    - Brain hemorrhage
    - Stroke

Epilepsy
- A disorder where the victim experiences repeated and unpredictable seizures.
- Unlike most other seizures or convulsions that can be traced to a particular cause, the cause of epileptic seizures is unknown.

Grand Mal Seizure
- A type of seizure where the victim may experience a warning sensation, and then possibly cry out, and then collapse into unconsciousness and experience violent muscle contractions.
- <u>A grand mal seizure has four phases:</u>

    1. **Aura**
        - The victim experiences sensations of taste, smell, or sound that are unusual and that serve to alert him that he is about to have a seizure.

    2. **Tonic Phase**
        - The victim loses consciousness and holds his breath, which causes him to appear cyanotic (having a bluish coloration of the skin). Also the victim's unconscious body becomes rigid with arms and legs fully extended.

    3. **Clonic Phase**
        - The victim experiences alternating muscle contractions and muscle relaxation, which cause the body to jerk. Occasionally the victim may urinate or defecate.

    4. **Postictal Phase**
        - The victim becomes comatose and the body goes limp. Eventually the victim returns to consciousness and experiences a sense of confusion, along with fatigue and headache.

7.2.2
Health Conditions of the Nervous System

- Spinal Stenosis
- Herniated Disk
- Sciatica
- Radiculopathy
- Achondroplasia
- Spondylolisthesis

Spinal Stenosis
- Spinal stenosis is a narrowing of spaces in the spine that results in pressure on the spinal cord and/or nerve roots.
- This disorder usually involves the narrowing of one or more of the following three areas of the spine:
    1. The canal in the center of the vertebral column through which the spinal cord and nerve roots run
    2. The canals at the base or roots of nerves branching out from the spinal cord
    3. The openings between the vertebrae through which nerves leave the spine and go to other parts of the body
- <u>This narrowing may</u>:
    - Affect either a small or large area of the spine.
    - Cause pressure to the lower part of the spinal cord, or to the nerve roots that branch out from that area, and possibly cause pain or numbness to the legs.
    - Cause pressure to the upper part of the spinal cord, and possibly cause pain to the neck, shoulders, or even the legs.
    - Include an array of symptoms that are not listed here.
- Spinal stenosis usually results from a gradual, degenerative aging process where either structural changes or inflammation can begin the process.

Herniated Disk
- A painful condition that results when a disk located between two vertebrae of the spine bulges backward, usually compressing a nerve root and interfering with the function of that nerve.

Sciatica
- Characterized by a pain that radiates down the sciatic nerve from a person's back into the buttocks and down the legs to the feet.

Radiculopathy
- Any disease that affects the spinal nerve roots.
- Symptoms include pain, numbness, tingling, and weakness.
- One possible cause of radiculopathy is a herniated disk.
- One possible symptom of radiculopathy is sciatica.

Achondroplasia
- It is a disorder of bone growth that results in the most common type of dwarfism.
- It occurs in one in every 15,000 to one in 40,000 live births.
- Most cases appear as spontaneous mutations.
- This means that 2 parents without achondroplasia may give birth to a baby with the condition.
- <u>It can also be inherited</u>.
- If a child gets the defective gene from 1 parent, the child will have the disorder.
- If 1 parent has achondroplasia, the infant has about a 50% chance of inheriting the disorder.
- If both parents have the condition, the infant's chances of being affected increase to about 75%.

Spondylolisthesis
- <u>When one vertebra slips forward on another</u>, which may result from a degenerative condition, or an accident, or, very rarely, may be acquired at birth.
- <u>When poor alignment of the spinal column causes a vertebra to slip forward onto the one below</u>, it can place pressure on the spinal cord or nerve roots at that point.

7.2.3

Arthritis Types That May Affect the Spine

- **Spondylosis**
- **Rheumatoid Arthritis**
- **Synovitis**
- **Spinal Stenosis**

Spondylosis
- If the degenerative process of <u>osteoarthritis</u> (see section 2.2.1) affects the facet joints and disks of the spine, the condition is sometimes referred to as *spondylosis*.
- This condition may be accompanied by disk degeneration and an enlargement or overgrowth of bone that narrows the central and nerve root canals.

Rheumatoid Arthritis
- The portions of the vertebral column with the greatest mobility (e.g., the neck area) are often the areas most affected in people with rheumatoid arthritis (see section 2.2.1).
- Rheumatoid arthritis is associated with inflammation and enlargement of the soft tissues (*synovium*) of the joints.

Synovitis
- Inflammation of the *synovial membrane*, which is the specialized connective tissue that lines the inner surface of capsules of synovial joints and tendon sheath.

Spinal Stenosis
- Although rheumatoid arthritis is not a common cause of spinal stenosis, the damage that results to the ligaments, bones, and joints begins as synovitis.

7.2.4

Acquired Causes of Spinal Conditions

- **Tumors of the Spine**
- **Trauma**
- **Paget's Disease**
- **Ossification of the Posterior Longitudinal Ligament**
- **Radiculopathy**
- **Lumbar Radiculopathy**
- **Cervical Radiculopathy**
- **Thoracic Radiculopathy**

Acquired conditions that cause spinal stenosis are the following:

Tumors of the Spine
- Abnormal growths of soft tissue that may affect the spinal canal directly by inflammation or by growth of tissue into the canal.
- Tissue growth may lead to bone resorption (bone loss due to over activity of certain bone cells) or displacement of bone.

Trauma
- Accidents may either dislocate the spine and the spinal canal or cause burst fractures that produce fragments of bone that penetrate the canal.

Paget's Disease
- A chronic disorder that typically results in enlarged and abnormal bones.
- Excessive bone breakdown and formation cause thick and fragile bone. As a result, bone pain, arthritis, noticeable bone structure changes, and fractures can occur.
- The disease can affect any bone of the body, but is often found in the spine. The blood supply that feeds healthy nerve tissue may be diverted to the area of involved bone.
- Also, structural problems of the involved vertebrae can cause narrowing of the spinal canal, producing a variety of neurological symptoms. Other developmental conditions may also result in spinal stenosis.

Ossification of the Posterior Longitudinal Ligament
- A condition that occurs when calcium deposits form on the ligament that runs up and down behind the spine and inside the spinal canal. These deposits turn the fibrous tissue of the ligament into bone. *Ossification* means "forming bone."
- These deposits may press on the nerves in the spinal canal.

Radiculopathy
- A pinched nerve in the spine resulting in discomfort and physical limitations.
- Caused by any disease that affects the spinal nerve roots.
- When there is compression of the spinal nerve roots, the symptoms include pain, numbness, tingling, and weakness.
- One of several possible causes of radiculopathy is a herniated disk.
- One of several possible symptoms of radiculopathy is sciatica, which is a condition that causes pain to radiate down from a person's back, to the buttocks, and then down the legs and into the feet.
- Radiculopathy is usually reversible with timely medical treatment.

- The types of radiculopathy specifically related to the areas of the spine where the nerves are compressed are the following:

    Lumbar Radiculopathy
    - Pressure on the nerve root in the lower back.
    - Can cause sciatica or intense pain in the legs.
    - Other symptoms include sexual dysfunction and incontinence.
    - In more severe cases, it can cause paralysis.

    Cervical Radiculopathy
    - Pressure on the nerve root in the neck.
    - It can cause painful burning or tingling in the neck, shoulders, and arms.

    Thoracic Radiculopathy
    - Pinched nerves in the center area of the spine.
    - This creates pain in the chest and torso area.
    - Occasionally the symptoms can be misdiagnosed as shingles.

7.2.5

Eye Conditions

- Cataract
- Astigmatism
- Keratoconus
- Blind Spot
- Legal Blindness
- Low Vision
- Hyperopia
- Myopia
- Presbyopia
- Dry Eye Syndrome
- Ghost Image
- Glare
- Halos
- Haze
- Eye Inflammation
- Keratitis
- Refractive Errors

Cataract
- A clouding of the lens in the eye that affects vision, most cataracts are related to aging.
- Cataracts are very common in older people. By age eighty, more than half of all Americans either have a cataract or have had cataract surgery.
- A cataract can occur in one eye or both eyes, but it cannot spread from one eye to the other.

Astigmatism
- When the surface of the cornea is not spherical, which causes a blurred image to be received at the retina.

Keratoconus
- A disorder characterized by an irregular corneal surface (cone shaped) resulting in blurred and distorted images.

Blind Spot
- Any gap in the visual field corresponding to an area of the retina where no visual cells are present. It is associated with eye disease.

Legal Blindness
- When visual acuity in the better eye with corrective lenses is 20/200 or worse, or when visual field is limited to a twenty-degree diameter (tunnel vision) or less in the better eye.
- A visual acuity of 20/200 requires that a person must be twenty feet or closer from an eye chart to see what a person with normal vision can see at two hundred feet.
- Note: These criteria are used to determine eligibility for government disability benefits as of this writing, and do not necessarily indicate a person's ability to function. Moreover, changes for government disability may occur at a later date.

Low Vision
- Visual loss that cannot be corrected with eyeglasses or contact lenses and interferes with daily living activities.

Hyperopia
- The condition otherwise known as farsightedness. It is the ability to see distant objects more clearly than close objects.
- May be corrected with glasses or contact lenses.

Myopia
- The condition otherwise known as nearsightedness, myopia is the ability to see close objects more clearly than distant objects.
- May be corrected with glasses or contact lenses.

Presbyopia
- The gradual loss of the eye's ability to change focus (*accommodation*) for seeing near objects caused by the lens becoming less elastic.
- Associated with aging and occurs in almost all people over age forty-five.

Dry Eye Syndrome
- A common condition that occurs when the eyes do not produce enough tears to keep the eye moist and comfortable.
- Common symptoms of dry eye include pain, stinging, burning, scratchiness, and intermittent blurring of vision.

Ghost Image
- A fainter second image of an object being viewed.

Glare
- Scatter from bright light that decreases vision.

Halos
- Rings around lights due to optical imperfections within or in front of the eye.

Haze
- The corneal clouding that causes the sensation of looking through smoke or fog.

Eye Inflammation
- The body's reaction to eye trauma, infection, or entrance of a foreign substance.
- Often associated with pain, heat, redness, swelling, and/or loss of eye function.

Keratitis
- Inflammation of the cornea.

Refractive Errors
- Imperfections in the focusing power of the eye (e.g., hyperopia, myopia, and astigmatism).

7.2.6

Eye Tests

- Dilation
- Fluorescein Angiography
- Refraction
- Tonometry
- Wavefront
- Diopter
- Snellen Visual Acuity Chart

Dilation
- To temporarily enlarge the pupil with special eye drops (*mydriatic*) to allow the eye care specialist to better view the inside of the eye.

Fluorescein Angiography
- A test to examine blood vessels in the retina, choroid, and iris.
- A special dye is injected into a vein in the arm and pictures are taken as the dye passes through blood vessels in the eye.

Refraction
- A test to determine the best eyeglasses or contact lenses to correct a refractive error (e.g., myopia, hyperopia, or astigmatism).

Tonometry
- The standard to determine the fluid pressure inside the eye (*intraocular pressure*).

Wavefront
- The measure of the total refractive errors of the eye, including nearsightedness, farsightedness, astigmatism, and other refractive errors that cannot be corrected with glasses or contacts.

Diopter
- The measurement of refractive error. A negative diopter value signifies an eye with myopia, and a positive diopter value signifies an eye with hyperopia.

Snellen Visual Acuity Chart
- One of many charts used to measure vision.

7.2.7

Eye Surgery and Treatments

- Ablate
- Ablation Zone
- Laser Keratome
- All-Laser LASIK (Bladeless LASIK)
- Excimer Laser
- Keratectomy
- Keratotomy
- Keratomileusis
- Laser
- LASIK
- Monovision
- Microkeratome
- Overcorrection
- Undercorrection
- Photo-Refractive Keratectomy
- Radial Keratotomy

Ablate
- A surgical term that means *to remove*.

Ablation Zone
- The area of tissue that is removed during laser surgery.

Laser Keratome
- A laser device used to create a corneal flap.

All-Laser LASIK (Bladeless LASIK)
- A procedure where a laser keratome device is used to cut a corneal flap for LASIK surgery.

Excimer Laser
- An ultraviolet laser used in refractive surgery to remove corneal tissue.

Keratectomy
- The surgical removal of corneal tissue.

Keratotomy
- A surgical incision of the cornea.

Keratomileusis
- The carving of the cornea to reshape it.

Laser
- The acronym for *light amplification by stimulated emission of radiation*.
- A laser is an instrument that produces a powerful beam of light that can vaporize tissue.

LASIK
- The acronym for *laser assisted in-situ keratomileusis*, which refers to creating a flap in the cornea with a microkeratome and using a laser to reshape the underlying cornea.

Monovision
- The purposeful adjustment of one eye for near vision and the other eye for distance vision.

Microkeratome
- A mechanical surgical device that is affixed to the eye by use of a vacuum ring. When secured, a very sharp blade cuts a layer of the cornea at a predetermined depth.

Overcorrection
- A complication of refractive surgery where the achieved amount of correction is more than desired.

Undercorrection
- A complication of refractive surgery where the achieved amount of correction is less than desired.

Photo-Refractive Keratectomy (PRK)
- A procedure involving the removal of the surface layer of the cornea (epithelium) by gentle scraping, and the use of a computer-controlled excimer laser to reshape the stroma.

Radial Keratotomy (RK)
- A surgical procedure designed to correct myopia (nearsightedness) by flattening the cornea using radial cuts.

CHAPTER 8

The Integumentary System

8.1 Anatomy of the Integumentary System · 373
    8.1.1   Skin · 375
    8.1.2   Skin Layers · 376
    8.1.3   Skin Cells · 378
    8.1.4   Exocrine Glands and Endocrine Glands · 379
    8.1.5   Sweat Glands · 382
    8.1.6   Mammary Glands · 383
    8.1.7   Ear Glands · 384
    8.1.8   Types of Hair · 385
    8.1.9   Hair Functions · 386
    8.1.10 Nails · 387

8.2 Integumentary System Injuries and Conditions · · · · · · · · · · · · · · · 389
    8.2.1   Skin Conditions · 391
    8.2.2   Common Adverse Skin Reactions · 394
    8.2.3   Burns · 395
    8.2.4   Types of Skin Wounds · 396
    8.2.5   Bleeding · 397
    8.2.6   Symptoms · 398
    8.2.7   Types of Blisters · 400
    8.2.8   Scar Tissue · 401
    8.2.9   Ear Condition · 402
    8.2.10 Hair and Scalp Conditions · 403
    8.2.11 Cosmetic Surgery · 404

8.1 Anatomy of the Integumentary System

8.1.1

Skin

- The largest organ of the body, skin represents about 7 percent of the body's weight.
- It is a dynamic protector between the body and its surrounding environment.
- It protects the body from disease, external injury, and the environment.
- The skin also helps to maintain normal body function and homeostasis.
- Social recognition, especially facial, is another function of the skin, as well as the expressions that enable us to consciously or unconsciously communicate.

8.1.2

Skin Layers

- **Epidermis**
- **Dermis**
- **Hypodermis**

Anatomy of human skin

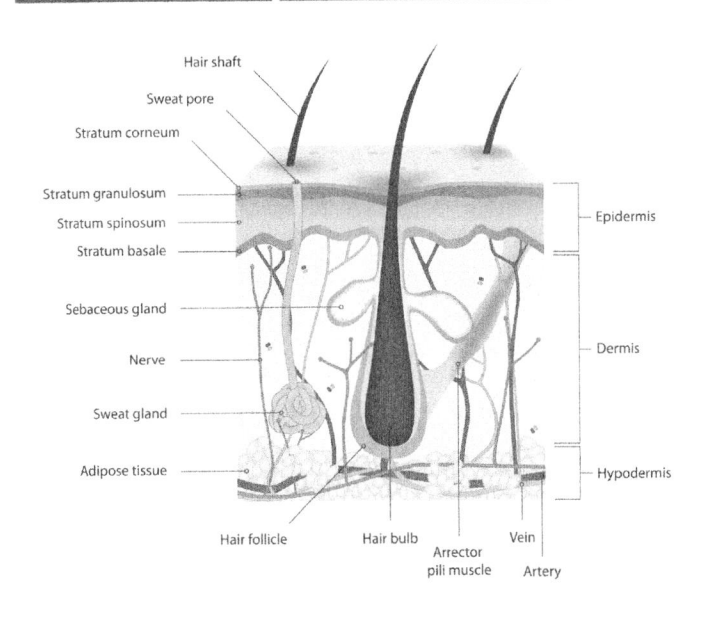

- Hair shaft
- Sweat pore
- Stratum corneum
- Stratum granulosum
- Stratum spinosum
- Stratum basale
- Sebaceous gland
- Nerve
- Sweat gland
- Adipose tissue
- Hair follicle
- Hair bulb
- Arrector pili muscle
- Vein
- Artery
- Epidermis
- Dermis
- Hypodermis

Epidermis
- The protective <u>outermost layer</u> of the skin that has between four and five sublayers. It is comprised of stratified squamous epithelium cells.

Dermis
- The <u>middle layer</u> of the skin that consists of two sublayers. It is comprised of the following:
    - Smooth muscle fibers
    - Connective tissues fibers
    - Blood vessels
    - Glands
    - Nerve endings
    - Hair follicles

Hypodermis (Subcutaneous)
- The <u>deepest layer</u> of the skin that is comprised of the following:
    - Fibrous connective tissues
    - Adipose tissue
    - Blood vessels
    - Lymph vessels

8.1.3

Skin Cells

- **Collagen**
- **Melanin**
- **Keratin**

Collagen
- A protein that is both tough and fibrous, and it is the most common structural protein in the body.
- An essential part of the bones, tendons, and connective tissues.
- The body uses collagen to help in holding its tissues and cells together, and to help tissues withstand stretching.

Melanin
- The dark pigment in the skin cells that is primarily responsible for skin color.
- Also found in hair, the pigmented tissue underlying the iris of the eye, and the *stria vascularis* of the inner ear.
- Brain tissues that contain melanin are the medulla and the pigment-bearing neurons.

Keratin
- A fibrous structural protein in the outer layer of the skin cells that is primarily responsible for strengthening the skin, waterproofing the skin, and protecting the skin cells from damage or stress.

8.1.4

Exocrine Glands and Endocrine Glands

- **Epithelial Tissues**
- **Glands**
- **Exocrine Glands**
- **Endocrine Glands**
- **Endocrine System**
- **Glands That Are Both Exocrine and Endocrine**
- **Hormones**

Epithelial Tissues
- <u>One of the four main tissue types</u> and widespread throughout the body.
- Form the covering of all body surfaces, line body cavities and hollow organs, <u>and are the major tissue in glands</u>.
- Perform a variety of functions that include protection, secretion, absorption, excretion, filtration, diffusion, and sensory reception.

Glands
- <u>Refers to organs that make one or more substances</u> in the body, such as hormones, digestive juices, sweat, tears, saliva, or milk.
- There are <u>two types of glands</u> in the human body:
    - *Exocrine Glands*
    - *Endocrine Glands*

See the definitions of these two terms on the next page.

Exocrine Glands
- Glands that produce and secrete substances <u>into ducts or openings that go to the inside or outside of the body.</u>
- Examples of these glands are:
    - *sweat glands* (see section 8.1.5 below)
    - *mammary glands* (see section 8.1.6 below)
    - *ear glands* (see section 8.1.7 below)
    - *salivary glands*
    - *mucous glands*
    - *lacrimal glands* (tear glands that constantly moisten, lubricate, and protect the surface of the eye)
    - *sebaceous glands* (they produce oily or waxy matter called *sebum*, to lubricate and waterproof the skin and hair. Sebum production and secretion is regulated by sex hormones. If a blockage occurs in these glands, they can become infected and result in acne)
- Many exocrine glands are associated with the digestive system.

Endocrine Glands
- Glands that produce and secrete substances directly into the bloodstream.
- Examples of these glands are:
    - *pituitary*
    - *pancreas*
    - *adrenal*
    - *hypothalamus*
    - *thyroid*
    - *parathyroid*
    - *pineal* (produces melatonin, a serotonin-derived hormone that modulates sleep patterns)
    - *testes*
    - *ovaries*

Endocrine System
- A system of endocrine glands and cells that make hormones that are released directly into the blood and travel to tissues and organs all over the body.
- The endocrine system controls:
    - *growth*
    - *sexual development*
    - *sleep*
    - *hunger*
    - *the way the body uses food*

Glands That Are Both Exocrine and Endocrine
- The liver and pancreas are both exocrine and endocrine glands.
- They are exocrine glands because they secrete bile and pancreatic juice into the gastrointestinal tract through a series of ducts, and endocrine glands because they secrete other substances directly into the bloodstream.

Hormones
- One of many substances made by glands.
- Hormones circulate in the bloodstream and control a vast number of functions of certain cells or organs.

8.1.5

Sweat Glands

- **Sudoriferous**
- **Eccrine**
- **Apocrine**

Sudoriferous Glands
- The sudoriferous sweat glands are located deep within the skin and throughout the entire body.
- Their primary function is to regulate body temperature by secreting perspiration onto the surface of the skin.
- The two main types of sudoriferous sweat glands are:

  1. *Eccrine*
     - The secretions of the eccrine sweat glands are not odor producing.
     - Primarily located in the skin of the back, palms, forehead, and soles of the feet.

  2. *Apocrine*
     - The secretions of the apocrine sweat glands are odor producing.
     - Primarily located in the skin of the pubic area and armpit area.

8.1.6

Mammary Glands

- A unique type of sudoriferous gland located inside the breasts.
- Their functionality occurs only during a woman's childbearing years.

8.1.7

Ear Glands

- **Ceruminous Glands**
- **Cerumen**

Ceruminous glands
- Secrete earwax (*cerumen*), which helps to protect the ear.

Cerumen
- Acts as an insect repellent and helps to keep the eardrum pliable.

8.1.8

Types of Hair

- **Lanugo**
- **Angora**
- **Definitive**

Lanugo
- Is fine and silky and found on the fetus in the last trimester. Its purpose is not fully understood.

Angora
- This type of hair grows continuously, such as on the scalp, or on the face of males once they have reached puberty.

Definitive
- This type of hair only grows to a certain length and then stops. Examples are eyelashes, eyebrows, armpit hair (*axillary*), and pubic hair.

8.1.9

Hair Functions

- The primary role of hair is to offer protection to certain areas of the body. For example, hair on the scalp and eyebrows offer protection against sunlight, and hair of the eyelashes and in the nostrils protect against airborne debris.

- Another function of hair is that it is a major component of social identity, expression, sexual attraction, and much more.

8.1.10

Nails

- **Fingers and Toes**
- **Nail Strength and Health**

Fingers and Toes
- The main purpose of nails is for the protection of the fingers and toes and to assist the fingers in picking up small items.
- The average growth rate of a healthy nail is about one inch every twenty-five weeks.

Nail Strength and Health
- Eating calcium-rich foods, gelatin, or any other nutrient, whether it is food or a supplement, does not improve nail health or nail growth. In fact, nails are not made of calcium; they are made of protein and extra amounts of protein do not help either.
- Nail polish can damage your nails. The chemicals used to make nail polish can cause your nails to become irritated and to split.

8.2 Integumentary System Injuries and Conditions

8.2.1

Skin Conditions

- **Dermatitis**
- **Erythema**
- **Acne**
- **Pustule**
- **Melanoma**
- **Boil**
- **Carbuncle**
- **Psoriasis**
- **Eczema**
- **Seborrhea**
- **Gangrene**
- **Athlete's Foot**
- **Hives**
- **Wart**
- **Shingles**
- **Nevus**

Dermatitis
- Inflammation of the skin.

Erythema
- Redness of the skin.

Acne
- Inflammation of the sebaceous glands.
- More common during puberty and adolescence because it is affected by *gonadal hormones* (the *gonads* are the sex glands; the testes in men and the ovaries in women).
- The most common locations for the pimples and blackheads of acne are on the face, chest, and back.

Pustule
- A small, localized pimple that contains pus.

Melanoma
- A cancerous tumor in the skin.

Boil (Furuncle)
- A localized bacterial infection that begins in a skin gland or hair follicle.

Carbuncle
- A localized bacterial infection that begins in a skin gland or hair follicle.
- Similar to a boil, except that it affects tissue of the subcutaneous layer.

Psoriasis
- A skin disease characterized by inflammation and circular, scaly patches of skin.

Eczema
- A noncontagious skin condition where there may be redness, blistering, oozing, and itching. Also the skin may be scaly, crusty, brownish, or thickened.

Seborrhea
- A skin disease characterized by overactive sebaceous glands, resulting in dandruff and oily skin.

Gangrene
- Death (*necrosis*) of body tissue caused by a loss of blood supply.
- There are two types of gangrene, wet and dry.
- Wet gangrene is a bacterial infection of the tissue and the gangrene can spread.
- Dry gangrene is absent of infection by bacteria and the gangrene does not spread.

Athlete's Foot (*Tinea Pedis*)
- A condition of the foot where a fungal disease is present in the skin.

Hives (*Urticaria*)
- Red eruptions on the skin that are usually accompanied by excessive itching.
- Usually the result of stress or allergic reactions.

Wart
- Skin growths caused by a viral infection in the top layer of the skin.
- Warts are noncancerous.

Shingles (*Herpes Zoster*)
- Inflammation of a nerve that results in blisters on the skin.
- Caused by the same virus as chicken pox.
- Symptoms include localized pain, fatigue, or headache.

Nevus
- A mole or a birthmark on the skin.

8.2.2

Common Adverse Skin Reactions

- **Blister**
- **Callus**
- **Corn**
- **Bedsores**

Blister
- A pocket of fluid that is located between the two top layers of skin, the epidermis and the dermis.
- Usual causes are burns and excessive friction resulting from rubbing against an object or the grasping of an object (e.g., the rubbing of the heel of the foot against the back of a tight shoe or using a shovel).
- See section 8.2.7 for more.

Callus
- A build-up of the outer layer of skin tissue (*stratum corneum*) as the body's way to adapt to frequent, excessive friction.

Corn
- A small callus on the foot.

Bedsores (*Decubitus Ulcer*)
- May develop on the skin of people who are bedridden for extended periods of time.

8.2.3

Burns

- First Degree
- Second Degree
- Third Degree

Burns
- Lesions affecting the skin as a result of heat or fire, sun exposure, electricity, or chemicals.
- There are <u>three classifications of burns</u>:

First Degree
- A burn that causes redness to only the epidermis (the upper layer of skin).

Second Degree
- A burn that causes blisters and involves the deeper layers of the epidermis and also the dermis.

Third Degree
- A burn that causes serious damage to all layers of the skin and also to underlying tissues, which may include muscle, bone, and other tissues that lie beneath the skin.

8.2.4

Types of Skin Wounds

- **Abrasion**
- **Avulsion**
- **Incision**
- **Laceration**
- **Puncture**

Abrasion
- An injury that results in the scraping away of a section of skin or mucous membrane.

Avulsion
- The type of wound that results in the forcible separation or tearing away of tissue from the body.

Incision
- A cut into the skin, usually occurring from a sharp object.

Laceration
- A cut or tear to the body tissue in a jagged or irregular pattern.

Puncture
- A small hole in the body tissue when a sharp object has pierced the skin.

8.2.5

Bleeding

- **Hemorrhage**
- **Hemarthrosis**
- **Hematoma**
- **Contusion**
- **Ecchymosis**

Hemorrhage
- Bleeding to a part of the body.

Hemarthrosis
- A hemorrhage occurring in a joint.

Hematoma
- A hemorrhage occurring in a muscle or tendon.

Contusion (Bruise)
- Slight bleeding under the skin as a result of injury, but in which the skin has not been broken.

Ecchymosis
- The purple discoloration that occurs from a contusion (bruise).

8.2.6

Symptoms

- **Inflammation**
- **Swelling**
- **Effusion**
- **Edema**

Inflammation
- The body tissue's response to an injury or medical condition, regardless of the cause.
- The signs and symptoms of inflammation may include any or all of the following:
    - Swelling
    - An increase of temperature at the site of the injury
    - Redness
    - Pain
    - Loss of function of the affected area

  <u>None of these symptoms should ever be ignored.</u>

Swelling
- An accumulation of fluids within the body as a result of disease or injury.

Effusion
- The loss of fluid into a body part.

Edema
- The swelling that occurs as a result of fluid accumulating in a body part.

8.2.7

Types of Blisters

Blister (Vesicle)
- A volume of fluid just beneath the outer layer of the skin, usually resulting in a raised oval or circular shape.
- Usual causes are burns, sunburns, or friction.
- This fluid acts to protect the damaged area, is usually sterile, and comes from a serum that seeps out from the blood vessels that are located in underlying layers of skin.
- Never attempt to burst a blister due to damage or injury because it could result in an infection to the area.

Other Causes of Blisters
- Certain skin conditions, such as *eczema* or *impetigo*, also cause blisters. In other cases, blisters are caused by viral infections such as chicken pox, herpes, and shingles.
- In these diseases, the blister may contain infectious viruses that can infect other people.
- Never attempt to burst a blister due to disease because it could result in an infection to the area and be infectious to other people.

Large Blisters (*Bullae*)
- Blisters that are more than a half-inch in diameter.
- If the blister worsens or its cause is unexplainable, consult with your physician.

8.2.8

Scar Tissue

- Hypertrophic Scar Tissue
- Keloid Scar Tissue
- Adhesions

Scar Tissue
- Any mark that is left on damaged tissue after the regular healing process has occurred.
- Scar tissue not only occurs on the skin, but on internal wounds as well.
- Scar tissue is an inelastic, tough, and fibrous protein collagen, which covers the site of the damage.
- The three main types of scars are the following:

Hypertrophic Scar Tissue
- A large, unattractive scar that can result from a wound that was infected.

Keloid Scar Tissue
- A large, irregularly shaped scar that continues to grow after the wound has healed.

Adhesions
- A type of scar tissue that forms between the parts of internal organs that had become separated.

8.2.9

Ear Condition

Tinnitus
- A condition that causes persistent or intermittent ringing sounds in one or both ears. These sounds may also be described as humming or buzzing.

8.2.10

Hair and Scalp Conditions

- **Alopecia**
- **Dandruff**

Alopecia
- Loss of hair, baldness.

Dandruff
- Common dandruff is when the scalp's outermost layer of skin cells flake off. Washing and brushing the hair keeps this condition under control.
- Abnormal dandruff is due to skin disease, such as *seborrhea* and *psoriasis*.

8.2.11

Cosmetic Surgery

- **Rhinoplasty**
- **Mentoplasty**
- **Mammoplasty**
- **Blepharoplasty**
- **Dermabrasion**

Cosmetic surgery
- Serves to improve a person's appearance or to correct physical abnormality.

Rhinoplasty
- Cosmetic surgery of the nose.

Mentoplasty
- Cosmetic surgery of the chin.

Mammoplasty
- Cosmetic surgery of the breasts.

Blepharoplasty
- Cosmetic surgery of the eyelids.

Dermabrasion
- Cosmetic surgery of the skin by removing the surface layers.

CHAPTER 9

Tissue Cell Abnormalities

9.1 Tissue Cell Abnormalities ·· 407
    9.1.1 Cancer Conditions ·· 409
    9.1.2 Body Types and Growth Abnormalities ···················· 414

9.1 Tissue Cell Abnormalities

9.1.1

Cancer Conditions

- **Cancer (Malignancy)**
  - *Carcinoma*
  - *Sarcoma*
  - *Leukemia*
  - *Lymphoma*
  - *Multiple Myeloma*
  - *Central Nervous System Cancer*
	- **Colon Cancer**
	  - *Adenocarcinoma*

- **Cancer Stages**	- **Colon Polyp**

- **Tumor (Neoplasm)**
  - *Malignant Tumor*
  - *Benign Tumor*
  - *Dysplasia*
	- **Skin Cancer**
	  - *Melanoma*
	  - *Basal Cell Carcinoma*
	  - *Squamous Cell Carcinoma*
	  - *Neuroendocrine Carcinoma*

- **Neuroblastoma**	- **Bronchial Adenoma**

- **Breast Cancer**
  - *Ductal Carcinoma*
  - *Lobular Carcinoma*
	- **Leukemia**

- **Prostate Cancer**	- **Lymphoma**
	  - *Hodgkin Lymphoma*
	  - *Non-Hodgkin Lymphoma*

Cancer
- A term for diseases in which abnormal cells divide without control and can invade nearby tissues. Also called *malignancy*.
- Cancer cells can also spread to other parts of the body through the blood and lymph systems.
- There are several main types of cancer:
    - *Carcinoma* is a cancer that begins in the skin or in tissues that line or cover internal organs.
    - *Sarcoma* is a cancer that begins in bone, cartilage, fat, muscle, blood vessels, or other connective or supportive tissue.
    - *Leukemia* is a cancer that starts in blood-forming tissue, such as the bone marrow, and causes large numbers of abnormal blood cells to be produced and enter the blood.
    - *Lymphoma* and *multiple myeloma* are cancers that begin in the cells of the immune system.
    - *Central nervous system cancers* are cancers that begin in the tissues of the brain and spinal cord.

Cancer Stages
- The extent of a cancer in the body.
- Staging is usually based on the size of the tumor, whether lymph nodes contain cancer, and whether the cancer has spread from the original site to other parts of the body.

Tumor
- The abnormal mass of tissue that develops when cells in a specific area multiply at an abnormal rate. Also called *neoplasm*.
    - *Malignant Tumor*: A cancerous tumor that can spread to other parts of the body. For example, lymphoma is a malignant tumor of the lymphoid tissue.
    - *Benign Tumor*: A tumor that is not cancerous.
    - *Dysplasia*: Cells that look abnormal under a microscope but are not cancer.

Neuroblastoma
- A type of cancer that forms from immature nerve cells. It usually begins in the adrenal glands but may also begin in the abdomen, chest, or in nerve tissue near the spine.
- Neuroblastoma most often occurs in children younger than five years of age. It is thought to begin before birth. It is usually found when the tumor begins to grow and cause signs or symptoms.

Breast Cancer
- The most common type of breast cancer is *ductal carcinoma*, which begins in the lining of the milk ducts (thin tubes that carry milk from the lobules of the breast to the nipple).
- Another type of breast cancer is *lobular carcinoma*, which begins in the lobules (milk glands) of the breast.
- Invasive breast cancer is breast cancer that has spread from where it began in the breast ducts or lobules to surrounding normal tissue.
- Breast cancer occurs in both men and women, although male breast cancer is rare.

Prostate Cancer
- A type of cancer that forms in tissues of the prostate (a gland in the male reproductive system found below the bladder and in front of the rectum).
- Prostate cancer usually occurs in older men.

Colon Cancer
- A type of cancer that forms in the tissues of the colon (the longest part of the large intestine).
- Most colon cancers are *adenocarcinomas* (cancers that begin in cells that make and release mucus and other fluids).

Colon Polyp
- An abnormal growth of tissue in the lining of the bowel. Polyps are a risk factor for colon cancer.

Skin Cancer
- A cancer that forms in the tissues of the skin.
- There are several types of skin cancer:
    - Skin cancer that forms in melanocytes (skin cells that make pigment) is called *melanoma*.
    - Skin cancer that forms in the lower part of the epidermis (the outer layer of the skin) is called *basal cell carcinoma*.
    - Skin cancer that forms in squamous cells (flat cells that form the surface of the skin) is called *squamous cell carcinoma*.
    - Skin cancer that forms in neuroendocrine cells (cells that release hormones in response to signals from the nervous system) is called *neuroendocrine carcinoma* of the skin.
- Most skin cancers form in older people on parts of the body exposed to the sun or in people who have weakened immune systems.

Bronchial Adenoma
- A cancer that forms in tissues of the bronchi (large air passages in the lungs including those that lead to the lungs from the windpipe).

Leukemia
- Characterized by an abnormal increase of white blood cells in the bone marrow.
- Since all blood cells originate in the bone marrow, the increase of leukemic cells interferes with the production of red blood cells, platelets, and normal white blood cells as these healthy cells are crowded out from the marrow.

Lymphoma
- A cancer that begins in cells of the immune system.
- There are two basic categories of lymphomas:
    - *Hodgkin lymphoma*, which is marked by the presence of a type of cell called the Reed-Sternberg cell.
    - *Non-Hodgkin lymphoma*, which includes a large, diverse group of cancers of immune system cells.
- Non-Hodgkin lymphomas can be further divided into cancers that have an *indolent* (slow-growing) course and those that have an *aggressive* (fast-growing) course. These subtypes behave and respond to treatment differently.
- Both Hodgkin and non-Hodgkin lymphomas can occur in children and adults, and prognosis and treatment depend on the stage and the type of cancer.

9.1.2

Body Types and Growth Abnormalities

- **Somatotype**
- **Aplasia**
- **Achondroplasia**
- **Dwarfism**
- **Ectomorph**
- **Macrosomia**
- **Gigantism**
- **Mesomorph**
- **Endomorph**

Somatotype
- Refers in general to body type.

Aplasia
- A limited or reduced growth in the development of body tissue or of any organ. Examples of aplasia are certain birth defects that result in stunted limbs. Another example is the reduced growth of bone marrow.

Achondroplasia
- This is the most common of the approximately two hundred types of dwarfism.

Dwarfism
- A condition characterized by a relatively normal-sized trunk and abnormally short arms and legs. Dwarfs typically reach an adult height of approximately four feet.

Ectomorph
- This is one of the three main classifications for human body types.
- A body that has many of the following traits characterizes the ectomorph:
    - Tends to be tall and slim
    - Tends to have a delicate build
    - Tends to have slight muscularity
    - Tends to have slower muscle growth
    - Tends to be relatively linear in shape
    - Tends to have narrow hips and pelvis
    - Tends to have small bones and joints
    - Tends to have trouble gaining weight.
    - Tends to have long arms and legs limbs
    - Tends to have less fat and muscle mass

Macrosomia
- A body that is significantly large with arms, legs, and head that are in proportion to the trunk.

Gigantism
- Excessive body growth, both in height and certain body parts.
- Disorders of the pituitary gland are responsible for this condition.
- It is important to note that this excessive body growth occurs during childhood or adolescence.

Mesomorph
- This is the second of the three main classifications for human body types.
- A body that has many of the following traits characterizes the mesomorph:
    - Tends to have muscular, hard body
    - Tends to develop muscle easily
    - Tends to have straight shoulders and good posture
    - Tends to have rectangular-shaped body
    - Tends to have thick bones
    - Tends to have thick skin
    - Tends to gain or lose weight easily

Endomorph
- This is the third of the three main classifications for human body types.
- A body that has many of the following traits characterizes the endomorph:
    - Tends to have a soft body
    - Tends to have underdeveloped muscles
    - Tends to have trouble losing weight
    - Tends to gain weight easily
    - Tends to add weight to the hips, buttocks and stomach areas
    - Tends to have a round shape
    - Tends to have small to medium bones
    - Tends to have short limbs in relationship to the entire body.

Quick Reference to Four Popular Anatomy Categories

1. Parts of the Body
2. Anatomical Positions
3. Bone and Cartilage Terms
4. Anatomical Numbers

1. Parts of the Body

Brachium	Relating to the arm
Cardio-	Relating to the heart
Cephalo-	Relating to the head
Dermo-	Relating to the skin
Hemo-	Relating to the blood
Myo-	Prefix that relates to muscle
Thorac-	Relating to the chest
Cervical	Relating to the neck
Lumbar	Relating to the lower back
Plantar	Sole, or bottom of the foot
Dorsal	Top surface of the foot or hand
Palmer	Palm surface of the hand

2. Anatomical Positions

Supra-	*Above*
Infra-	*Below*
Superior	*Toward the head*
Inferior	*Away from the head*
Anterior or Ventral	*Toward the front of the body*
Posterior or Dorsal	*Toward the back of the body*
Medial	*Toward the center, or midline, of the body; the opposite of lateral*
Lateral	*Away from the center, or midline, of the body the opposite of medial*
Proximal	*The direction that is toward the attached end of a limb, closest to the head*
Distal	*The direction that is away from the attached end of a limb, furthest from the head*
Superficial	*An external location; found close to or on the body surface*
Deep	*An internal location, further beneath the body surface than superficial structures*

3. Bone and Cartilage Terms

Oste- Relating to bone

Origin The bone that <u>remains relatively stationary when the muscle attached to it contracts</u> to create a body movement. The origin is often, but not always, the proximal bone.

Insertion The bone that <u>moves when the muscle attached to it contracts</u> to create a body movement. The insertion is often, but not always, the distal bone.

Articulation The connection point or joint between bones, or between bones and cartilage

Arthro- Relating to a joint

Chondro- Relating to the cartilage

Costo- Relating to the ribs

Ilio- Relating to the ilium

Cervical Vertebrae Seven bones in the spine's neck region

Thoracic Vertebrae Twelve bones in the spine's middle back region

Lumbar Vertebrae Five bones in the lower back region

4. Anatomical Numbers

Bi- *Two*

Tri- *Three*

Medical Terms

- **Diagnosis**
- **Prognosis**
- **Risk Factor**
- **Primary Risk Factor**
- **Acute**
- **Chronic**
- **Idiopathic**
- **Stenosis**

Diagnosis
- A physician's determination of the cause of a person's disease, illness, or injury.

Prognosis
- A physician's determination of the probable course and outcome of a person's disease, illness, or injury.
- Any prognosis is no more than an informed prediction and may be proven wrong over a period of time.

Risk Factor
- A particular characteristic associated with an individual that makes that individual predisposed to a medical condition or disease. These characteristics include, but are not limited to, inherited traits, acquired conditions, diseases, behavioral patterns, or any other characteristic that increases one's vulnerability to a medical condition or disease.

Primary Risk Factor
- The particular characteristic that is directly associated with a major health problem. A typical example of a primary risk factor is smoking, because it is a direct cause of lung cancer.

Acute
- A symptom or condition that has a very sudden onset.
- Acute conditions are not always severe, and they usually do not last for a long time.
- Acute is the opposite of chronic.

Chronic
- A symptom or condition that continues over a long period of time.
- Chronic is the opposite of acute.

Idiopathic
- Conditions that have no known cause.

Stenosis
- A condition that refers to the narrowing, or decrease in diameter of
    - a tubular organ, such as a blood vessel;
    - the intestine;
    - the spine;
    - a canal;
    - a duct; or
    - any other bodily passage system.

The Four Main Types of Body Tissues

- **Muscle Tissue**......................See Section 1.1.2
- **Connective Tissue**............See Section 1.1.11
- **Nerve Tissue**......................See Section 7.1.1
- **Epithelial Tissue**...............See Section 8.1.4

GLOSSARY

Achilles Tendon: a powerful tendon that attaches both the *gastrocnemius* and the *soleus* muscles to the heel.

Adenosine Triphosphate (ATP): one of the body's two high-energy storage compounds.

Alkalosis: an excessively alkaline condition of the body fluids or tissues that may cause weakness or cramps.

Areolar: a common type of loose connective tissue that is the most widely distributed type of connective tissue in the body.

Arthralgia: joint pain

Body Dysmorphic Disorder: a psychological condition where a person suffers from a distorted perception of the body, resulting in the belief that his or her body, or a part of the body, is painfully ugly. Examples include perceptions of the face, nose, breasts, or muscle size and shape.

Bronchodilator: a type of drug that is inhaled and causes small airways in the lungs to open up. They are used to treat breathing disorders, such as asthma or emphysema.

Chondromalacia: means "soft cartilage." In this condition, the articular cartilage gets soft and becomes diseased.

Coracoacromial Arch: a narrow bony space that is located at the top of the shoulder.

Creatine Phosphate (CP): one of the body's two high-energy storage compounds.

Crepitus: the grating, crunching, or creaking sound heard when the cartilage around joints erodes and the surfaces in the joint grind against one another (as in osteoarthritis or rheumatoid arthritis), or when the fractured surfaces of two broken bones rub together.

Dysphonia: trouble with the voice when trying to talk, including hoarseness and change in pitch or quality or voice.

Dysplasia: cells that look abnormal under a microscope but are not cancer.

Emesis: the medical term for vomiting

Erythrocytes: red blood cells

Exocrine Glands: organs that make substances such as sweat, tears, saliva, or milk. These glands release the substances into a duct or opening to the inside or outside of the body.

Fascicle: a bundle of skeletal muscle fibers surrounded by perimysium.

Hydrolysis: refers to a chemical reaction that must include water wherein one chemical compound produces another compound.

Hypokinesis: a lack of energy or a lack of activity

Iliotibial Band (ITB): a thick structure of fascia that extends down across the lateral (outside) section of the knee.

Islets (or Islands) of Langerhans: located in the pancreas and they produce the hormone insulin.

Lactate: responds to aerobic and anaerobic exercises by fueling the muscles, delaying fatigue, and preventing injury.

Lactic Acid: converts pyruvate into lactate to fuel the muscles.

Leukocytes: white blood cells

Myocyte: a muscle fiber, or muscle cell, within the muscle.

Myoglobin: an oxygen-binding protein found in the heart and skeletal muscles. There, it attaches to oxygen to provide extra energy for muscle cells. However, when the heart or skeletal muscle is injured, myoglobin is released into the blood. Myoglobin blood tests are used to diagnose the extent of injury, as in a heart attack.

Nucleus: the structure in a cell that contains the chromosomes. The nucleus has a membrane around it, and is where RNA is made from the DNA in the chromosomes.

Ossification: to form bone

Plantar Fasciitis: an inflammation of the *plantar fascia*, which is the primary supportive soft tissue that comprises the sole of the foot.

Platelets: see *Thrombocytes*

Prone: when the body is lying flat on the stomach, face down.

Pyogenic: pus-producing

Pyruvate: an intermediate compound in the metabolism of carbohydrates, proteins, and fats.

Range of Motion: to the distance and direction a joint can move between the flexed position and the extended position.

Resistive Force: external force that resists the motion of another force.

Sarcolemma: the plasma membrane of skeletal muscle and cardiac muscle cells.

Sepsis: a dangerous condition where there is the presence of bacteria or their toxins in the blood or tissues.

Supine: when the body is lying flat on the back, face up.

Synthesis: when two or more chemical compounds, or chemical elements, combine to form a more complex compound.

Systemic Disease: a disease that affects a number of organs and tissues, or affects the body as a whole.

Therapeutic Angiogenesis: the use of genes to grow new blood vessels to repair or replace damaged blood vessels in the heart muscle.

Thrombocytes: commonly known as blood platelets, which stop bleeding at the site of a damaged vessel by binding together to form a clot. Thrombocytes (platelets) are produced in red bone marrow.

Valsalva Maneuver: an increase in intrathoracic pressure and blood pressure caused by holding one's breath while lifting heavy weight. Exhaling through the mouth when lifting is a way to avoid this problem.

Vasovagal Reaction: the result of standing up too suddenly. It causes dizziness and a fainting sensation related to a sudden lowering of heart rate and blood pressure.

Vegans: people who include plant sources in their diets. A strict vegan does not eat any food that comes from an animal source.

Vegetarian, Lacto-ovo: people who include dairy products and eggs in their diets but exclude meat, fish, and poultry.

Vegetarian, Lacto: people who include dairy products in their diets.

Vegetarian, Ovo: people who include eggs in their diets.

Vegetarian, Pesco: people who include dairy products, eggs, and also fish in their diets.

Vegetarian, Semi: people who include dairy products, eggs, fish, and also chicken in their diets.

INDEX

Charts are indicated by "c" following page numbers.
Figures and diagrams are indicated by "f" following page numbers.

A

AA (arachidonic acid), 212
Abdominals
    breathing using abdominal muscles, 311
    exercises targeting, 183
    external oblique, 8f, 31c
    increasing definition (getting six-pack), 184
    internal oblique, 31c
    muscle strength exercises. *See* Core exercises
    primary joint motions, 31c
    rectus abdominis, 8f, 31c
    skeletal muscles of, 31c
    transverse abdominis, 31c
    workout chart, 180c
Abduction, 89
    arm, 33c
    hip, 27c, 31c
    shoulder, 26c, 33c
    wrist, 35c
Ablate, 367
Ablation zone, 367
Abrasion, 396
Abscesses, 127
Accommodation (vision), 349, 363
Achilles tendon, 62, 425
Achilles tendonitis and rupture, 62
Achondroplasia, 357, 414
Acid–base balance, 145

Acid reflux, 129–130
ACL (anterior cruciate ligament) tears, 64
Acne, 220, 380, 391
Actin, 13, 17
Acuity (vision), 350, 363
Acute promyelocytic leukemia, 220
Adam's apple (epiglottis), 37, 303f, 304, 306
Addison's disease, 156, 187
Adduction, 88
    hip, 27c
    pectoralis major, 33c
    scapula, 32c
    shoulder, 26c
    wrist, 35c
Adductor brevis, 27c
Adductor longus, 8f, 27c
Adductor magnus, 27c
Adenosine triphosphate (ATP), 13, 161, 162, 167, 425
Adhesions, 401
Adipose tissue, 137, 376f, 377
Adrenal glands, 380
Adrenaline (epinephrine), 163
Aerobic exercises
    ATP production from, 167
    beginner guidelines, 264–270
        age as factor, 267
        boredom factor, 268, 270
        calisthenics, 267

cardiorespiratory training methods, 268
circuit training, 269
conditioning exercise program, 266
conditioning progression plan, 266
continuous training method, 268
cool-down phase, 270
cross training (composite training), 270
duration of workouts, 265, 267, 281
Fartlek training, 269
frequency of workouts, 264, 267, 268
heart rate chart, 265c
improvement conditioning stage, 267
initial conditioning stage, 267
intensity, 264, 267–269, 277, 281
intermediate slow distance, 268
interval training, 269
long slow distance, 268
maintenance conditioning stage, 268, 270
stretching, 265, 267
warm-ups, 265, 266
benefits of, 158
capacity to consume oxygen, 263
compared to weight lifting
adding muscle, 158
calorie burning, 147
definition of, 167
dynamic (ballistic) stretches, 46
in fitness program, 140
injuries and conditions common to
Achilles tendonitis and rupture, 62
patellar tendonitis (jumpers knee), 63
torn meniscus (cartilage), 64
Karvonen Formula (also known as Heart Rate Maximum Reserve Method), 275–279
submaximal aerobic exercise, 275
training heart rate range (THRR), 273
types of, 147
warm-ups and cool-downs, 181–182, 265, 266, 270
warning for working out at or near 90 percent of maximum heart rate, 281
Aerobic glycolysis, 11
Aerophagia, 319
Age. *See also* Childhood and infancy
acne most common in puberty, 391
beginner aerobic exercise guidelines, 267
BMI underestimating body fat in elderly persons, 169
body building program, clearance after age 50, 178
body composition and, 136
cataracts in older people, 362
coenzyme Q10 (CoQ10), decrease with aging, 229
Crohn's disease, age of onset, 126

exercise program, clearance after age 50, 280
facial hair growth in males, 385
free radicals' role in aging process, 228
metabolism, decline in, 158, 159
muscle loss as people age, 203
neuroblastoma in children under age 5, 411
presbyopia as part of aging process, 363
prostate cancer in older men, 411
skin cancer more likely in older people, 412
strength gain, best age for, 17
stroke, increasing risk with age, 296
training heart rate chart by age, 265c
training heart rate range (THRR) related to age, 273–274
Aggressive cancer, 413
Agonist muscle, 21–22, 41, 45, 46, 50
AI (adequate intake), 196
Air sacs, 307. *See also* Alveoli
Airways, 304, 305
Alanine, 206
Albumin, 115
Alcoholic withdrawal, seizures caused by, 353
Algal oils, 212
Alimentary canal, 107
Alkalosis, 186, 319, 425
All-Laser LASIK (Bladeless LASIK), 367
All-trans-retinoic acid (ATRA), 220
Alpha-linolenic acid (LNA), 212

Alpha-tocopherol (vitamin E), 217, 218, 224, 228
ALS (amyotrophic lateral sclerosis), 68
Alveolar ducts, 304, 307, 308
Alveolar sacs, 308
Alveoli, 303f, 304, 307–309, 312, 317, 318
Amenorrhea, 143
Amino acids, 115, 193, 204, 205–206
    essential amino acids, 205–206
    nonessential amino acids, 205–206
Amitotic, 334
Amyotrophic lateral sclerosis (ALS), 68
Anaerobic activity
    in aerobic conditioning exercise program, 266
    anaerobic threshold, 168
    definition of, 167
    muscle fiber, 10
Anaerobic ATP, 13, 162
Anaerobic glycolysis, 10
Anal fissures, 127
Anatomical numbers, 420
Anatomical planes, 86, 87f
Anatomical positions, 418
Anemia, 221, 223, 288
Angora (hair type), 385
Ankles
    dorsiflexion, 28c, 90
    flexion, 28c
    flexor digitorum longus, 30c
    flexor hallucis longus, 30c
    plantar flexion, 28c, 90
    plantaris, 30c
    popliteus, 30c

posterior tibialis, 30c
primary joint motions, 30c
skeletal muscles, 30c
soleus, 30c
sprains, 61
synovial joint motions, 25, 28c, 91c
synovial joints, 85
Anorexia nervosa, 143
Antagonist muscle, 21–22, 41, 45, 46, 50
Anterior chamber (eyes), 344f, 345
Anterior cruciate ligament (ACL) tears, 64
Anterior (front) deltoids, 26c, 33c
Anterior position, 418
Anterior tibial artery, 258f
Anterior tibialis, 8f, 28c, 30c
Antioxidants, 228–229. See also Vitamins
  phytochemicals (plant chemicals) as, 230
Anus, 108f, 109, 112
  hemorrhoids, 124
Anvil (ear), 81
Aorta, 237f, 239, 242f, 255
Apex of the heart, 248
Apical pulse site, 248
Aplasia, 414
Appendicular skeleton, 75, 79
Appendix, 108f, 109, 112
Aqueous fluid (aqueous humor), 344, 345
Arachidonic acid (AA), 212
Areolar (tissue), 425
Arginine, 206
Armpits, sweat glands in, 382

Arms. See also Biceps; Elbows; Shoulders; Tendonitis; Triceps; Wrists
  abduction, 33c
  brachium, 417
  lateral rotation, 33c
  medial rotation, 33c
  primary joint motions, 35c
  pronation, 34c, 35c, 90
  raising above head, pain caused by, 58
  rotation motion, 59. See also Rotator cuffs
  skeletal muscles, 35c
  supination, 34c, 90
  workout chart, 180c
Arrector pili muscle, 376f
Art awareness, 332f
Arteries, 236, 237f, 239. See also Aorta
  anterior tibial arteries, 258f
  arteriosclerosis (thickening/hardening of arteries), 286
  ateriloes, 255
  atherosclerosis (thickening/hardening of arteries), 286, 287
  basilar artery, 258f
  brachiocephalic artery, 242f
  capillaries, 255
  carotid arteries, 248, 255, 258f
    left common carotid artery, 242f
  compared to veins, 255
  coronary arteries, 237f, 255
  coronary artery disease (CAD), 287
  diagram of, 255f
  elastic layer, 255f

femoral artery, 258f
function of, 255
hardening of arteries, 286, 287
iliac artery, 258f
inner layer, 255f
left subclavian artery, 242f
outer layer, 255f
posterior tibial arteries, 258f
pulmonary arteries, 255, 258f, 310
    left pulmonary artery, 237f, 242f, 256
    right pulmonary artery, 237f, 242f
radial arteries, 248, 258f
skin and, 376f, 377
smooth muscle, 255f
superficial temporal arteries, 248
venous system, 255
Arthralgia, 425
Arthritis, 95–98, 358
    ankylosing spondylitis, 97
    diagram comparing normal joint to osteoarthritis, 96f
    gout, 98
    infective arthritis, 98
    osteoarthritis, 96f, 97, 358
    rheumatoid arthritis, 97, 358
    seronegative arthritis, 97
    Still's disease, 97
Arthro- (body part designation), 419
Arthroscopic surgery, 64
Articulations, 84, 419
Ascending aorta, 237f
Ascorbic acid (vitamin C), 217, 218, 223, 228
Asparagine, 206

Aspartic acid, 206
Aspirin, peptic ulcer caused by, 121
Asthma, 318, 425
Astigmatism, 362
Aterioles, 255
Atherosclerosis, 286, 287
    risk for stroke, 296
Athletes' daily requirements, 204
Athlete's foot (tinea pedis), 392
ATP (adenosine triphosphate), 13, 161, 162, 167, 425
ATRA (all-trans-retinoic acid), 220
Atrial natriuretic peptide, 155
Atrioventricular (mitral) valve, 242f
Atrioventricular (tricuspid) valve, 242f
Atrophy, 18, 144
Auditory ossicles, 78, 80
Auscultation, 245
Autoimmune diseases, 97
Autonomic nervous system, 155, 328–329
    parasympathetic nervous system, 329
    sympathetic nervous system, 329
Avocados, 210
Avulsion, 396
Axial skeleton, 75, 78
Axillary hair, 385
Axons, 333f, 334
    demyelination of, 335
    unmyelinated and myelinated, 335

B

Back
    latissimus dorsi, 8f, 9f, 21, 32c
    synovial joint motions, 26c

workout chart, 180c
low back pain, 57
lower back vertebrae. See Lumbar vertebrae
lumbar, 417
middle back vertebrae. See Thoracic vertebrae
rhomboids, 9f, 32c, 89
sweat glands, 382
trapezius muscles, 8f, 9f, 32c, 89
    lower trapezius, 32c
    middle trapezius, 32c
    upper trapezius, 32c
workout chart, 180c
Bacteria
    gangrene spread by, 392
    in mouth, 113
"Bad" cholesterol. See LDL
"Bad" fats, 213
Balance, 331
Baldness, 403
Ball & socket joint, 91c
Ballistic (dynamic) flexibility, 42, 46
Ballistic (dynamic) stretches, 46, 48
Barley, 201
Baroreceptors, 155
Basal cell carcinoma, 409c, 412
Basal metabolic rate (BMR), 7, 142, 159–160
Baseball players, shoulder impingement syndrome, 58
Basilar artery, 258f
Basketball players, injuries and conditions common to
    Achilles tendonitis and rupture, 62

ACL tears, 64
dynamic (ballistic) stretches, 46
patellar tendonitis (jumpers knee), 63
Beats per minute (bpm), 249
Bedsores (decubitus ulcer), 394
Beginner aerobic exercises, 264–270. See also Aerobic exercises
Bench press. See Body building
Benign tumor, 409c, 411
Beriberi, 221
Beta-carotene, 218, 228
Bi- (anatomical number two), 420
Biceps, 8f. See also Biceps brachii; Brachialis; Brachioradialis
    concentric contractions of, 29
    primary joint motions, 34c
    skeletal muscles, 26c
Biceps brachii, 26c, 34c
Biceps curls, 19, 21, 88, 180, 180c
Biceps femoris, 9f, 27c, 28c, 30c
Biceps tendon rupture, 58
Bile, 115
Bile acids, 289
Binge eating, 146
Binocular vision, 349
Biomechanical problems, 63
Biotin (vitamin B-7), 217, 218, 222
Birth defects. See Congenital conditions; Fetus
Birthmark, 393
Blackheads. See Acne
Bleeding, 397. See also Blood clotting
    vitamin K deficiency causing, 224
Blindness. See Vision

Blind spot, 345, 363
Blinking, 23
Blisters (vesicles), 394, 400
Blood. *See also* Red blood cells; White blood cells
    amount in body, 251
    anemia. *See* Anemia
    color of, 253
    components of, 252–253
    conditions, 288
    cyanosis, 288
    function, 251
    hemo-, 417
    hemoglobin, 251, 253, 288
    pH regulation, 301
    plasma, 251, 252
    platelets, 251, 252
Blood cell production, 75
Blood circulation cycle, 235, 238, 242*f*
Blood clots
    hemorrhoid complications, 125
    vitamin E preventing, 224
Blood clotting
    ability of blood to clot, 251
    calcium's role, 225
    circulatory system assisting in, 235
    liver's role, 115
    platelets' role, 252
    vitamin K's role, 224
Blood infection, 98
Blood pooling, methods to avoid, 182, 270
Blood pressure, 247. *See also* High blood pressure; Low blood pressure
    calcium's role, 225
    diastolic blood pressure, 246, 247
    heat exhaustion, 186
    magnesium's role, 226
    regulation of, 154, 155
    sphygmomanometer to measure, 245
    systolic blood pressure, 246, 247
    warm-up and cool-down to prevent sudden drop, 181–182, 270
    white coat hypertension, 247
Blood-sodium level, 187
Blood sugar levels, regulation of, 154, 155, 165. *See also* Glucose; Insulin
    glycemic index, 202
    magnesium's role, 226
    Vitamin B-6's help with, 222
Blood vessels, 14*f*, 236, 254–257. *See also* Arteries; Veins
    avascular system, 257
    brain, rupture in. *See* Stroke
    conditions, 295–296
        aneurysm, 295
        cerebral embolism, 295
        cerebral hemorrhage, 295
        cerebral thrombosis, 295
        cerebrovascular accident (CVA), 295
        stroke, 295–296
    diagram of, 255*f*
    repairing damage of, 251, 257
    therapeutic angiogenesis, 257
    types of, 254
    vascular system, 257
    visceral muscle in, 7

Blurred vision, 57
BMR (basal metabolic rate), 7, 142, 159–160
Body building, 175–188. See also Weight lifting
   abdominal definition (building six-pack), 184
   adding muscle, 151, 158
   biceps tendon rupture, 58
   body sculpting, 148
   burning calories from. See Calories
   effective methods for, 177
   endorphins produced by, 163
   heat conditions, 185–187. See also Heat conditions
   increasing weight used in, 178
   osteoporosis, training to address, 188
   spot reducing exercises, 183
   technique, 178
   theory of, 177
   warm-ups and cool-downs, 181–182
   Wolff's Law, 188
   workout chart, 180c
Body composition, 133–173. See also Energy production and sources
   adipose tissue, 137
   analysis of, 136
   body fat, 136, 137, 149
      BMI to estimate, 169
      burning calories while at rest, 150
      understanding percentages, 173

   body function stabilization, 154–155
   body mass index (BMI), 169
      formula, 170–171
      range chart for weight categories, 172c
   brown fat cells, 138
   burning calories. See Calories
   caloric intake, reduction of, 139
   cellulite, 137
   chemical imbalances, 156–157
   determining, 149
   eating disorders, 143–146. See also Eating disorders
   energy balance theory, 152
   exercise for weight loss, 140
   fat cells, types of, 138
   food as energy, 152
   high blood-potassium level (hyperkalemia), 156
   homeostatis, 154, 155
   hyperkalemia, 156
   hyperthyroidism, 157
   hypokalemia, 156
   hypothyroidism, 157
   lean body mass, 136, 137
      determining, 149
      muscle size's effect on, 149
   low blood-potassium level (hypokalemia), 156
   metabolism. See Metabolism
   overfat as preferred term, 172
   set-point theory, 152
   stabilization process, 154–155
   subcutaneous fat, 137

thermal effect of food (TEF), 153
visceral fat, 137
weight, 135–136
    stabilization, 152–153
weight loss, methods for, 135, 139–140. *See also* Weight loss
white fat cells, 138
Body dysmorphic disorder, 425
Body fat, 136, 137, 149
  BMI to estimate, 169
  burning calories while at rest, 150
  understanding percentages, 173
Body function stabilization, 154–155
Body image, distortion of, 143
Body mass index (BMI), 169
  formula, 170–171
  range chart for weight categories, 172c
Body sculpting, 148
Body temperature, regulation of, 154, 155
  circulatory system's role in, 235
  inflammation at site of injury, 398
  sweat gland's role in, 382
  water's role in, 198
Body tissue, types of, 423
Body types and growth abnormalities, 414–416. *See also* Dwarfism
  achondroplasia, 414
  aplasia, 414
  ectomorph, 415
  endomorph, 416
  gigantism, 415
  macrosomia, 415
  mesomorph, 416
  somatotype, 414
Body weight. *See* Body composition
Boil (furuncle), 392
Bone marrow, 75, 252, 253
  cancers starting in, 409c, 410, 413
Bones. *See also* Joints; Skeletal system
  bone loss, 359
  calcium's role in formation of, 225. *See also* Calcium
  categories of, 75
  copper's role in formation of, 226
  cranium, 78, 80
  dislocation, 56
  ears, 81
  face, 81
  fluoride's role in formation of, 226
  functions of, 75
  hips, 79
  hyperthyroidism's effect on, 157
  muscle contractions, 18
  normal joint vs. osteoarthritis, 96f
  origin (proximal bone), 419
  Paget's disease, 360
  phosphorus's role, 227
  proximal bone, 419
  skeletal muscles attached to, 7, 14f, 75
    distal, 20
    proximal, 20
  stationary bone in muscle contraction, 419
  stress fracture, 61, 99
  terminology, 419
  Vitamin A's protective powers, 220
  vitamin K's protective powers, 224

Wolff's Law, 188
Bone spur, 96f
Boredom factor in exercising, 268, 270
Borg, Gunnar, 272
Borg Scale, 272
Boron, 218, 225
Bowel blockage, 127
Bowel movements. See also
    Constipation; Diarrhea; Irritable
    bowel syndrome (IBS)
    hemorrhoids, causes of, 124
Boxers' risk of concussion, 57
BPM (beats per minute), 249
Brachialis, 26c, 34c
Brachiocephalic artery, 242f
Brachioradialis, 8f, 26c, 34c
Brachium, 417
Bradycardia, 285
Brain
    brain stem, 330f
    in central nervous system, 325, 327
    cerebellum, 330f, 331
    cerebrum, 330f, 331
    corpus callosum, 330f, 331
    energy requirements of, 331
    functions of, 327, 332f
    hypoglycemia's effect on, 166
    hypothalamus, 330f
    injuries and conditions
        concussion, 57
        hemorrhage, 353
        oxygen deprivation, 331, 353
        ruptured vessel in. See Stroke
        seizures as result of, 353
    testing for abnormal brain waves (EEG test), 336
    vitamin B-9 deficiency causing defects, 223
    left brain functions, 332f
    medulla, 330f, 331, 378
    midbrain, 330f
    oxygen needed by, 331
    parts of (diagram), 330f
    pituitary gland, 155, 330f, 380
    pons, 330f
    right brain functions, 332f
    ventricles, 330f
    weight of, 331
Brain stem, 330f
Brain waves, 336
Bread, 201, 223
Breakfast, importance of, 142
Breast cancer, 409c, 411
Breasts
    mammary glands, 379, 383
    mammoplasty, 404
Breathing. See also Respiratory system
    abnormalities, 319
    adrenaline's effect on, 163
    aerophagia, 319
    autonomic nervous system controlling, 328
    BMI as factor for problems, 169
    gastroesophageal reflux disease (GERD) and respiratory problems, 130
    hyperventilation, 319
    hypochloremia symptom of breathing difficulty, 186

hypokalemia, symptom of shallow breathing for, 156
medulla controlling, 331
muscles used for, 311–313
nervous system impairment causing breathing difficulty, 325
into paper bag, 319
valsalva maneuver, 319
Bronchi (singular bronchus), 303f, 304, 307–309
Bronchial adenoma, 409c, 412
Bronchial asthma, 318
Bronchial tree, 304, 308
Bronchioles, 303f, 304, 307, 309
Bronchitis, 317, 318
Bronchodilator, 425
Brown fat cells, 138
Brown sugar, 201
Bruising, 397
vitamin K deficiency causing, 224
Bulimia, 146
Bullae (large blisters), 400
Burning calories. See Calories
Burns, 395
blisters, 394, 395, 400
Bursa, 56, 84
bursitis, 56, 58
defined, 84
pinching injury (shoulder impingement), 58
Bursitis, 56, 58
Butter, 209, 213, 289. See also Dairy products
Buttocks
gluteus maximus, 9f, 31c
gluteus medius, 8f, 31c
gluteus minimus, 31c
primary joint motions, 31c
skeletal muscles, 31c
workout chart, 180c

C

Calcium, 75, 218, 219, 224, 225
Calisthenics, 267
Callus, 394
Calories, 191
Calorie (with capital "C"), 191
calorie burning
by adding muscle, 147–148, 150–151, 158
exercise comparison of, 147–148
definition of, 191
empty calories, 194
intake reduction, 139. See also Diet
kilocalorie, 191
large calorie, 191
to lose one to two pounds per week, 141
in main nutrient groups, 192
measuring energy from, 152
per meal, 142
saturated fat intake, 215
small calorie, 191
total fat intake, 215
Calves, 30c
Cancer, 409–413. See also specific types of cancer
aggressive course, 413
basal cell carcinoma, 409c, 412

benign tumor, 409c, 411
BMI as factor for, 169
breast cancer, 409c, 411
bronchial adenoma, 409c, 412
carcinoma, 409c, 410
central nervous system cancers, 409c, 410
coenzyme Q10 (CoQ10) effects, 229
colon cancer, 409c, 412
colon polyp, 409c, 412
definition of, 410
ductal carcinoma, 409c, 411
dysplasia, 409c, 411
free radicals' role, 228
Hodgkin lymphoma, 409c, 413
indolent course, 413
leukemia, 220, 409c, 410, 413
lobular carcinoma, 409c, 411
lung cancer, 422
lymphoma, 409c, 410, 411, 413
malignancy, 409c, 410, 411
melanoma (skin cancer), 392, 409c, 412
multiple myeloma, 409c, 410
neoplasm, 409c, 411
neuroblastoma, 409c, 411
neuroendocrine carcinoma, 409c, 412
non-Hodgkin lymphoma, 409c, 413
prostate cancer, 409c, 411
sarcoma, 409c, 410
skin cancer, 392, 409c, 412
squamous cell carcinoma, 409c, 412
stages of, 410
tumor (neoplasm), 409c, 411
types (chart), 409c
vitamin A and vitamin A acid as cancer preventative/treatment, 220
vitamin B-1 facilitating growth of cancer cells, 221
vitamin B-2 levels in cancer patients, 221
vitamin B-3 as cancer preventative/treatment, 221
vitamin B-7 as cancer preventative/treatment, 222
vitamin B-12 as cancer preventative/treatment, 223
vitamin E as cancer preventative/treatment, 224
Candy, 201
Canola oil, 210, 212
Capacity to consume oxygen, 263
Capillaries, 255, 307, 310, 312
Caracobrachialis, 26c
Carbohydrates, 139, 152, 161, 195, 199–202. *See also* Starch; Sugar
    calories per gram, 192, 199
    chromium's role with, 226
    complex carbohydrates, 200
        digestion of, 201
        food examples, 201
    conversion to triglycerides, 213
    definition of, 199
    disaccharides, 199
    food examples, 201
    glycemic index, 202
    manganese's role with, 226
    monosaccharides, 199
    phosphorus's role with, 227

polysaccharides, 200
simple carbohydrates, 199
digestion of, 201
food examples, 201
suggested daily intakes, 197
Carbon, 207
Carbon dioxide
cardiovascular system removing, 235
red blood cells transporting, 253
respiration, 302, 305, 307, 309, 312, 313, 319
in veins, 257
Carbuncle, 392
Carcinoma, 409c, 410
Cardiac arrest
dangers of, 238
fish oil's omega-3 fatty acids protecting against, 212
hyperkalemia symptom, 156
Cardiac arrhythmias, 285
hyperkalemia symptom, 156
hypokalemia symptom, 156
warm-up and cool-down preventing, 181–182
Cardiac asthma, 318
Cardiac muscle, 6f, 7, 240
muscle force, 18
myocarditis, 287
sarcolemma, 12f, 13
Cardio- (body part designation), 417
Cardiopulmonary endurance, 262
Cardiopulmonary system, 235. See also Circulatory system
Cardiorespiratory endurance, 262
Cardiorespiratory training methods, 268

Cardiovascular endurance, 262
Cardiovascular system, 235. See also Circulatory system
Carotid arteries, 248, 255, 258f
Carotid pulse site, 248
Carpals, 77f, 79, 91c
Cartilage, 37
chondro- (body part designation), 419
disks. See Disks
elastic cartilage, 37
fibrocartilage, 37
hyaline cartilage, 37
injuries and conditions
chondromalacia, 425
chondromalacia patella, 62
normal joint vs. osteoarthritis, 96f
torn cartilage (meniscus), 37, 64
meniscus/menisci, 37, 64
terminology, 419
types of, 37
Cartilaginous joints (synchondroses), 85
Catalysts, enzymes acting as, 114
Cataracts, 362
free radicals causing, 228
Cauda equina, 341
Cecum, 108f, 109, 112
Cells. See also Red blood cells; White blood cells; *other specific types of cells*
dysplasia, 426
vitamin E protecting, 224
Cellular metabolism, 302
Cellular respiration, 302

Cellulite, 137
Central nervous system, 325, 327
    cancers starting in, 409c, 410
    muscle contraction, 13
    oligodendrocytes, 335
Central nervous system cancers, 409c, 410
Central retinal artery, 345
Central retinal vein, 345
Central vision, 350
Cephalo- (body part designation), 417
Cerebellum, 330f, 331
Cerebrum, 330f, 331
Cervical (body part designation), 417
Cervical radiculopathy, 361
Cervical vertebrae, 82f, 83, 419
Cheese. See Dairy products
Chemical imbalances, 156–157
Chest
    muscles (pectoralis major), 8f, 21, 33c
    synovial joint motions, 26c
    workout chart, 180c
    thorac- (designator), 417
Chicken pox, 393, 400
Childhood and infancy
    excessive body growth during (gigantism), 415
    neuroblastoma in children under age 5, 411
    Still's disease (arthritis), 97
    Type 1 diabetes, 165
    zinc's role, 227
Chin, cosmetic surgery for (mentoplasty), 404
Chloride/Chlorine, 218, 219, 225

Cholecalciferol (vitamin D), 217, 218, 224
Cholesterol, 208, 209, 215, 221, 289–294. See also HDL; LDL
    characteristics of, 289
    cholesterol/HDL ratio, 292c
    dangerous levels of, 289
    definition of, 289
    dietary fat and cholesterol levels, 293–294
    effects of eating less cholesterol, 293
    hypercholesterolemia, 288
    lipoproteins, 289, 290, 293
    range references, guidelines for, 292c
    recommended daily intake, 289
    sources of, 289, 294
    total blood cholesterol, 291, 292c
    triglycerides, 208, 212, 213, 291
Chondro- (body part designation), 419
Chondromalacia, 425
Chondromalacia patella, 62, 63
Choroid, 344f, 345
Chromium, 218, 226
Chromosomes, 334
Chronic obstructive pulmonary disease (COPD), 318
Chyme, 114
Cilia, 304, 306
Ciliary muscles, 346
Ciliary processes, 345, 346
Circuit training, 269
Circulatory system, 231–258. See also Blood pressure; Blood vessels; Heart; Lungs

components of, 235–236
diagnosing circulatory sounds, 245–246
  auscultation, 245
  Korotkoff sounds, 246
  sphygmomanometer, 245
  stethoscope, 245, 248
diagram of, 258f
medulla controlling, 331
pulse, 248
Circulatory system injuries and conditions, 283–296
blood conditions, 288
blood vessel conditions, 295–296
cholesterol. See Cholesterol
diabetes causing, 165
heart attacks. See Myocardial infarction
heart conditions. See Heart disease and conditions
hypoglycemia, 166
Circumduction, 90
Clavicle, 77f, 79
Clotting. See Blood clotting
Coagulation, 115
Cobalamin (vitamin B-12), 217, 218, 223
Coccyx, 82f, 83
Coconut oil, 209
Coenzyme Q10 (CoQ10), 229
Colitis, 122
  ulcerative colitis, 126
Collagen, 378
Colon, 108f, 109, 112
Colon cancer, 409c, 412
  Crohn's disease and, 128
Colonoscopy, 128

Colon polyp, 409c, 412
Color vision, 346
Coma. See also Unconsciousness
  heat stroke, 186
  high blood-sodium level (hypernatremia), 187
Complex carbohydrates, 200, 201
Compression, 67
  abdominals, 31c
Compulsive exercising, 144, 146
Concentric contractions, 19–20, 29
Concussion, 57
Conditioning exercise program, 266
Conditioning progression plan, 266
Condyloid (ellipsiod) joint, 91c
Cones (cone cells), 346
Confusion
  concussion, 57
  high blood-sodium level (hypernatremia), 187
  hyponatremia, 187
  stroke symptoms, 296
Congenital conditions
  aplasia, 414
  dwarfism, 357
  indirect inguinal hernia, 119
  Type 1 diabetes, 165
Conjunctiva, 346
Connective tissue, 36–37, 377, 423. See also Tendon
  flexibility of, 43
Consciousness, loss of. See Loss of consciousness
Constipation
  hemorrhoids, causes of, 124
  IBS with constipation (IBS-C), 122

445

Continuous training method, 268
Contractile proteins, 13, 17
Contractions. See Muscular system
Contrast sensitivity, 349
Contusion (bruise), 397
Convulsions. See Seizures
Cool-downs and warm-ups, 181–182, 265, 266, 270
COPD (chronic obstructive pulmonary disease), 318
Copper, 218, 219, 226
Coracoacromial arch, 58, 425
Core exercises, 57
Corn (foot), 394
Cornea, 344, 344f
Corn oil, 210, 212
Corn sweetener or syrup, 201
Coronary arteries, 237f, 255
 coronary artery disease (CAD), 287
Corpus callosum, 330f, 331
Cortisone injections, 56, 62, 63, 101
Cosmetic surgery, 404
Costo- (body part designation), 419
Coughing, 306, 317
 autonomic nervous system controlling, 328
CP (creatine phosphate), 162, 163, 425
Cramping. See Spasms
Cranium bones, 77f, 78, 80
Creatine phosphate (CP), 162, 163, 425
Creativity, 332f
Crepitus. See Grinding/crackling sound
Crohn's disease, 97
Crohn's disease, 126–128
Cross-country skiers, slow-twitch muscle fiber, 11

Cross training (composite training), 270
Cushing's syndrome, 156, 187
Cyanocobalamin, 217, 223
Cyanosis, 288, 318. See also Discoloration
Cysteine, 206

D

Dairy products, 201, 209, 213, 216
 cholesterol levels, 289, 294
 vitamin A in, 220
 vitamin B-12 in, 220
 vitamin D in, 224
Dancers engaging in compulsive exercising, 144
Dandruff, 392, 403
Death
 diabetes causing, 165
 emphysema causing, 318
 fish oil's omega-3 fatty acids protecting against sudden death, 212
 heat stroke, 186
 when playing sport due to myocarditis, 287
Decubitus ulcer (bedsores), 394
Deep position, 418
Definitive hair, 385
Dehydration, 144, 145
Déjà vu, seizures causing, 353
Deltoids, 8f, 9f, 33c
 anterior (front) deltoids, 26c, 33c
 middle deltoids, 26c, 33c
 posterior (rear) deltoids, 26c, 33c
Dematitis, 391
Demyelination, 335

Dendrites, 333f, 334
Depression (motion), 89
    scapula, 32c
Dermabrasion, 404
Dermis, 376f, 377
Dermo- (body part designation), 417
Descending aorta, 237f
Desserts, 201, 214
Dextrose, 201
DHA (docosahexaenoic acid), 212
Diabetes, 164, 165–166. *See also specific types below*
Diabetes insipidus, 187
Diabetes mellitus, 165
    hyperventilation caused by, 319
    stroke, increasing risk with, 296
Diagnosis, 421
Diagnostic tests and tools
    auscultation, 245
    Borg Scale, 272
    cholesterol range references, 292c
    dynamometer test, 68
    electrocardiogram (EKG), 286
    electroencephalogram (EEG), 336
    EMGs (electromyograms), 68
    ergometer, 261
    eye tests, 365–366
    goniometer test, 69
    inclinometer test, 69
    Korotkoff sounds, 246
    muscular injuries and conditions, 68–69
    palpation, 248
    sphygmomanometer, 245
    stethoscope, 245, 248
    stress tests, 261, 263, 271
    taking pulse, 248
Diaphragm, 303f, 311–313
    hiatal hernia and, 120
Diarrhea
    hemorrhoids caused by, 124
    hypochloremia caused by, 186
    hypokalemia caused by, 156
    hyponatremia caused by, 187
    IBS with diarrhea (IBS-D), 122
Diarthroses. *See* Synovial joints
Diarthrosis (muscles involved in synovial joint motions), 25
Diastolic blood pressure, 246, 247
Diet, 189–230. *See also* Water consumption
    amino acids. *See* Amino acids
    basal metabolic rate (BMR) factor, 159
    breakfast, importance of, 142
    calories. *See* Calories
    carbohydrates. *See* Carbohydrates
    cholesterol, effects of eating less, 293
    cholesterol in, 294
    coenzyme Q10 (CoQ10), foods containing, 229
    eating smart, 142
    empty calories, 194
    essential nutrients, 193
    exercise-related, 185
    fasting, 144
    fats. *See* Fat consumption
    fatty acids. *See* Fatty acids
    lipids, 208. *See also* Lipids
    to lose one to two pounds per week, 141

main nutrient groups, 192, 195
meat consumption, 213, 216. See also Meat consumption
for nail strength, 387
nutrient density, 194
plant foods, 210, 216. See also Plant foods
proteins. See Proteins
smaller and more frequent meals, 142
starches. See Starches
starvation, 145
suggested daily intakes, 197, 203, 212
symbols that express quantities of nutrients, 196
vitamin A, foods containing, 220
vitamin B-1, foods containing, 221
vitamin B-2, foods containing, 221
vitamin B-6, foods containing, 222
vitamin B-7, foods containing, 222
vitamin B-12, foods containing, 223
vitamin C, foods containing, 223
vitamin D, foods containing, 224
vitamin E, foods containing, 224
for weight loss, 139, 184
Digestive system, 105–115
alimentary canal, 107
anus, 108f, 109, 112
appendix, 108f, 109, 112
autonomic nervous system controlling, 328
calories used in digesting, absorbing, and metabolizing food, 153
cecum, 108f, 109, 112
chyme, 114
colon, 108f, 109, 112
conditions. See Digestive system injuries and conditions
duodenum, 108f, 109, 110
endocrine system's role, 381
enzymes, 113, 114
esophagus, 107, 108, 108f
gall bladder, 115
gastric juices, 114
gastrointestinal (GI) tract, 107–109, 108f
lower GI tract, 109
upper GI tract, 107–108
glands' role with, 380
hydrochloric acid's role, 225
ileum, 108f, 109, 111, 112
injuries. See Digestive system injuries and conditions
jejunum, 109, 110
large intestine, 108f, 109, 112
liver, 115. See also Liver
mouth, 107, 113. See also Mouth
pancreas, 115, 380. See also Pancreas
pharynx, 107, 114
ptyalin, 113, 114
rectum, 108f, 109, 112
saliva, 113. See also Saliva
salivary glands, 113, 114, 379, 380
small intestine, 108, 108f, 109, 110–111, 115
stomach, 107, 108, 108f
teeth, 114. See also Teeth

thermal effect of food (TEF), 153
Digestive system injuries and conditions, 117–130
    acid reflux, 129–130
    Crohn's disease, 126–128
    functional GI disorders, 122
    gastroesophageal reflux (GER), 129
    gastroesophageal reflux disease (GERD), 129
    hemorrhoids, 124–125
    hernia, 119–120
        femoral, 120
        hiatal, 120
        inguinal, 119
        umbilical, 120
    irritable bowel syndrome (IBS), 122–123
    peptic ulcer, 121
Dilation, 365
Diopter, 366
Direct inguinal hernia, 119
Disabled persons
    bedsores, 394
    benefits for legal blindness, 363
Disaccharides, 199
Discoloration
    cyanosis, 288, 318
    ecchymosis, 397
    in grand mal seizure, 354
    sprained ankle, 61
Disks (discs, correct spelling), 339
    bulging disk, 339f
    degenerative disk, 339f
    diagram of, 339f
    function of, 327, 338
    herniated disk, 339f, 356
        radiculopathy, 360
    herniation diagnosis, 68
    location of, 327, 338
    normal disk, 339f
    osteophyte formation in degeneration, 339f, 358
    ruptured disks, 57
    spondylosis, 358
    thinning disk, 339f
Dislocation, 56
Distal attachment, 20
Distal position, 418
Diuretics, 146
    hyponatremia, 187
Dizziness
    concussion, 57
    cool-down preventing, 182
    hyperventilation, 319
    stroke symptoms, 296
    vasovagal reaction, 428
    warm-up and cool-down preventing, 270
DNA, 13, 226, 427
    free radicals damaging, 228
    selenium's role, 227
    vitamins need for production of, 223
    zinc's role, 227
Docosahexaenoic acid (DHA), 212
Doctor consultation. See Physicians, consultation of
Dorsal (body part designation), 417
Dorsal position, 418
Dorsiflexion, 30c, 90

Drusen, 346
Dry eye syndrome, 364
Dry gangrene, 392
Ductal carcinoma, 409c, 411
Duodenum, 108f, 109, 110
    peptic ulcer, 121
    tumors, 121
Dwarfism, 357, 414, 415
Dynamic (ballistic) stretches, 46, 48
Dynamometer test, 68
Dysphonia, 426
Dysplasia, 409c, 411, 426
Dyspnea, 317

E

Ears
    bones in (auditory ossicles), 78, 80
    cerumen (earwax), 384
    ceruminous glands, 384
    elastic cartilage, 37
    stria vascularis of inner ear, 378
    tinnitus, 402
Eating disorders, 143–146
    anorexia nervosa, 143
    binge eating, 146
    bulimia, 146
    compulsive exercising, 144
    fasting, 144, 146
    ketosis, 145
    starvation, 143–145
    yo-yo effect, 146
Eating smart. See Diet
Eccentric contractions, 19
Ecchymosis, 397
Ectomorph, 415
Eczema, 392, 400

Edema, 319, 399
EEG (electroencephalogram), 336
Effusion, 399
Eggs
    cholesterol in, 289, 294
    vitamins in, 221–224
Eicosapentaenoic acid (EPA), 212
Ejection fraction, 250
EKG (electrocardiogram), 286
Elastic bandages, 67
Elastic cartilage, 37
Elastic property (or elastic elongation), 43
Elbows
    injuries and conditions
        bursitis, 56
        tennis elbow (epicondylitis), 58
        synovial joint motions, 25, 26c, 91c
        synovial joints, 85
Electrical burn, 395
Electrocardiogram (EKG), 286
Electrocardiograph, 286
Electroencephalogram (EEG), 336
Electrolyte imbalance, 144
Electromyograms (EMGs), 68
Elevation, 89
    of injured part above heart, 67
    scapula, 32c
Ellipsiod (condyloid) joint, 91c
Elongation, 41. See also Stretching
Emergency care for stroke, 296
Emesis. See Vomiting
EMGs (electromyograms), 68
Emphysema, 318, 319
    bronchodilator to treat, 425
Empty calories, 194

Endocardium, 240
Endocrine glands, 379–380
Endocrine system, 381
    hypothalamus's role in, 155
Endomorph, 416
Endorphins, 163, 182, 270
Endothelium, 348
Endoysium, 14f, 15
Endurance athletes
    protein supplements, 204
    slow-twitch muscle fiber, 11
Energy balance theory, 152
Energy production and sources
    adrenaline (epinephrine), 163
    BMR requirements, 159. *See also* Basal metabolic rate (BMR)
    brown fat cells and, 138
    burning calories. *See* Calories
    digestive process, 114
    endorphins, 163
    energy balance theory, 152
    enzymes. *See* Enzymes
    fat for. *See* Fat consumption
    food for, 152
    glucose for. *See* Glucose
    glycogens. *See* Glycogens
    insulin, 164
    ketosis, 145
    lactate (lactic acid), 164
    phosphagens, 162, 167
    substrate, 161
Enzymes, 163
    as antioxidants, 228
    calcium's role, 225
    definition of, 163
    digestive, 113, 114, 163
    manganese's role, 226
    molybdenum's role, 227
    in saliva, 113, 114
    vitamin B-1 helping with, 221
    vitamin B-3 helping with, 221
    vitamin B-6 helping with, 222
    vitamin B-7 helping with, 222
EPA (eicosapentaenoic acid), 212
Epicardium, 240
Epicondylitis (tennis elbow), 58
Epidermis, 376f, 377
Epiglottis (Adam's apple), 37, 303f, 304, 306
Epilepsy, 354
Epimysium, 14f
Epinephrine, 163
Epithelial tissues, 379, 423
Epithelium, 220, 348
Equilibrium, 331
Ergocalciferol, 224
Ergometer, 261
Erythema, 391
Erythrocytes. *See* Red blood cells
Esophagitis, 130
Esophagus, 107, 108, 108f, 305
    Barrett's esophagus, 130
    cancer of, 130
    inflamed, 130
    sphincter, hiatal hernia and, 120
    stricture in, 130
    ulcer in, 121
    visceral muscle in, 7
Essential amino acids, 205–206
Essential fatty acids, 211
Essential hypertension, 247
Essential minerals, 218

Essential nutrients, 193
Essential vitamins, 217
Estrogen use, increasing risk of stroke, 296
Ethmoid bone, 80
Eversion of foot, 30c, 90
Excimer laser, 368
Exercise. *See also specific type of exercise*
   aerobic workouts. See Aerobic exercises
   basal metabolic rate (BMR) factor, 159
   calorie burning comparison, 147–148
   compulsive exercising, 144
   decrease in, cause of muscle loss, 159
   diabetes, control of, 166
   heart healthy, 259–281
      beginner aerobic training guidelines, 264–270. *See also* Aerobic exercises
      Borg Scale, 272
      capacity to consume oxygen, 263
      cardio endurance, 262
      ergometer, 261
      Karvonen Formula (also known as Heart Rate Maximum Reserve Method), 275–279
      Max Cardiac Output, 263
      maximum heart rate and calculations, 273–274
      Max Oxygen Extraction, 263
      MET system, 271
      safe training, 280–281
      stress tests. *See* Stress tests
      talk test, 272
      training heart rate range (THRR), 273
      VO2 Max, 263
   importance of, 140, 142
   rowing machines, 261
   stationary bicycles, 261
   treadmills, 261
Exercise-induced asthma, 318
Exertion, rate of
   Borg Scale, 272
   stress tests. *See* Stress tests
   talk test, 272
Exhalation, 313
Exocrine glands, 379–380, 426
Extension, 88
   elbow, 26c
   hip, 27c, 31c
   knee, 28c, 30c
   shoulder, 26c, 32c
   wrist, 35c
Extensor carpi radialis, 9f, 35c
Extensor carpi ulnaris, 9f, 35c
Extensor digiti minimi, 8f
Extensor digitorum brevis, 8f
Extensor digitorum longus, 28c
Extensor hallucis brevis, 8f
External hemorrhoids, 124
External oblique, 8f, 31c
   workout chart, 180c
External respiration, 302
Eye conditions, 362–364
   astigmatism, 362
   blind spot, 363

cataracts, 362
dry eye syndrome, 364
eye inflammation, 364
farsightedness, 363
ghost image, 364
glare, 364
halos, 364
haze, 364
hyperopia, 363
keratitis, 364
keratoconus, 362
legal blindness, 363
low vision, 363
myopia, 363
nearsightedness, 363
presbyopia, 363
refractive errors, 364
surgeries and treatments, 367–369
    ablate, 367
    ablation zone, 367
    All-Laser LASIK (Bladeless LASIK), 367
    excimer laser, 368
    keratectomy, 368
    keratomileusis, 368
    keratotomy, 368
    laser, 368
    laser keratome, 367
    LASIK, 368
    microkeratome, 368
    monovision, 368
    overcorrection, 368
    photo-refractive keratectomy (PRK), 369
    radial keratotomy (RK), 369
    undercorrection, 369
tests for, 365–366
    dilation, 365
    diopter, 366
    fluorescein angiography, 365
    refraction, 365
    Snellen visual acuity chart, 366
    tonometry, 365
    wavefront, 366
Eye inflammation, 364
Eyelids, blepharoplasty for, 404
Eyes, 342–349. See also Vision
accommodation, 349, 363
acuity, 350, 363
anterior chamber, 344f, 345
aqueous fluid (aqueous humor), 344, 345
binocular vision, 349
blind spot, 345
central retinal artery, 345
central retinal vein, 345
choroid, 344f, 345
ciliary muscles, 346
ciliary processes, 345, 346
conditions, 362–364. See also Eye conditions
cones (cone cells), 346
conjunctiva, 346
contrast sensitivity, 349
cornea, 344, 344f
drusen, 346
endothelium, 348
epithelium, 348
fovea, 346
functions of, 349
fundus, 346
inferior rectus muscle, 344f

intraocular pressure (IOP), 349
    tonometry to determine, 365
iris, 344, 344f, 378
lacrimal gland, 346
lens, 344, 344f
macula, 345
optic cup, 347
optic disc (optic nerve head), 347
optic nerve, 344f, 345
parts of (diagram), 344f
peripheral vision, 350
photoreceptors, 346
posterior chamber, 347
pupil, 344, 344f
refractive power, 350
    refraction test for, 365
retina, 344f, 345
retinal pigment epithelium (RPE), 347
rods (rod cells), 347
Schlemm's canal, 347
sclera, 347
stroma, 348
superior rectus muscle, 344f
tests for. See Eye conditions
trabecular meshwork, 347
uvea (uveal tract), 345, 347
visual field, 350
vitreous gel, 344f
vitreous humor, 344, 347
zonules, 348

F

Facet joints, 340
Facial bones, 78, 81
Facial hair growth, 385
Facial recognition, 375
Fainting or feeling faint
    heat exhaustion, 186
    hypoglycemia, 166
    warm-up and cool-down preventing, 181–182, 270
Farsightedness, 363
Fartlek training, 269
Fascia, 36
    iliotibial band (ITB), 426
Fascicles, 14f, 15, 426
Fashion models engaging in compulsive exercising, 144
Fasting, 144, 146
Fast-twitch white muscle fiber, 10, 23
Fat. See Body composition
Fat absorption, 115
Fat cells
    functions of, 207
    types of, 138
Fat consumption, 139, 207–208. See also Cholesterol; Lipids
    "bad" fats, 213
    calories per gram, 192
    cholesterol levels and dietary fat, 293–294
    chromium's role with, 226
    eating foods with lower fat, 142
    energy production from, 152, 207
    fat as nutrient, 195, 207
    manganese's role with, 226
    phosphorus's role with, 227
    saturated fats, 197, 209–210
        intake, 215
    suggested daily intakes, 197, 215
    total fat intake, 215

triglycerides, 208, 212, 213, 291
Fat-free dairy products, 216
Fatigue
    in grand mal seizure, 354
    hypoglycemia, 166
    shingles (herpes zoster), 393
Fats. *See* Fat consumption
Fat-soluble vitamins, 207, 218, 220, 224, 291
Fatty acids, 161, 167, 193, 207, 209–212
    essential fatty acids, 211
    monounsaturated fatty acids, 210
    omega-3 polyunsaturated fatty acids, 210, 211–212
    omega-6 polyunsaturated fatty acids, 210, 211–212
    polyunsaturated fatty acids, 210
    saturated fatty acids, 209–210. *See also* Saturated fats and fatty acids
    trans fatty acids, 210, 214
Feces, 112
Feed and breed response, 329
Feet. *See also* Ankles; Tarsals
    Achilles tendon, 62, 425
    athlete's foot (tinea pedis), 392
    corns, 394
    dorsal, 417
    dorsiflexion, 90
    eversion motion, 30c, 90
    high arches increasing plantar fasciitis, 62
    injuries and conditions. *See also* Footwear problems
        plantar fasciitis, 62
        stress fracture, 99
    inversion motion, 30c, 90
    plantar, 417
    plantar flexion, 90
    posterior tibialis, 30c
    primary joint motions, 30c
    rheumatoid arthritis, 97
    skeletal muscles, 30c
    standard anatomical position, 76
    sweat glands in soles, 382
    synovial joint motions, 91c
Female vs. male. *See* Male vs. female
Femoral artery, 258f
Femoral hernia, 120
Femoral vein, 258f
Femur, 77f, 79
Fertility
    CoQ10's effect on, 229
    hyperthyroidism's effect on, 157
Fetus
    lanugo hair, 385
    vitamin B-9 deficiency causing defects in, 223
Fibrocartilage, 37
Fibrous joints (syndesmoses), 85
Fibula, 77f, 79
Fight or flight response, 329
Fingers. *See* Hands; Thumb motion
First-degree burns, 395
Fish, 212, 222, 224
Fish oils
    supplements, 212
    vitamin A in, 220
Fissures, 304, 308
Fistulas, 127
Flaxseed oil, 212
Flexibility, 42. *See also* Stretching

ballistic (dynamic) flexibility, 42, 46
of connective tissue, 43
range of motion, 42. See also Range
    of motion
static flexibility, 42, 45
Flexion, 88
    abdominals, 31c
    ankle, 28c
    elbow, 26c, 34c
    hip, 27c
    knee, 28c, 30c
    pectoralis major, 33c
    shoulder, 33c, 34c
    wrist, 35c
Flexor carpi radialis, 8f, 9f, 35c
Flexor carpi ulnaris, 35c
Flexor digitorum longus, 28c, 30c
Flexor hallucis longus, 28c, 30c
Fluid accumulation (edema), 319, 399
Fluid replacement. See Dehydration
Fluorescein angiography, 365
Fluoride, 218, 219, 226
Folic acid (vitamin B-9) (also called
    Folate), 217, 218, 223
Food
    diet. See Diet; *specific food types*
    digestion of. See Digestive system
    energy from. See Energy production
        and sources
Football players, injuries and conditions
        common to
    ACL tears, 64
    concussion risk, 57
Footwear problems
    Achilles tendonitis and rupture, 62
    plantar fasciitis, 62
Force
    muscle force, 18, 23
    resistive force, 19
    restive force, 428
Forearms. See Arms
Fovea, 346
Free radicals, 223, 224, 228
    antioxidants' protective role, 228
    phytochemicals' protective role, 230
    selenium's protective role, 227
Frontal bone, 80
Frontal (coronal) plane, 86, 87f
    motion on, 88–89
Frontal sinus, 303f, 304, 305
Front deltoids. See Anterior (front)
    deltoids
Fructose, 199, 201
Fruits and vegetables, 201, 212, 216, 223
    phytochemicals' role, 230
    vitamins from, 220–224
Fruit sugar (fructose), 199, 201
Functional GI disorders, 122
Fundus, 346
Fungus (athlete's foot), 392
Furuncle (boil), 392

G

g (grams), 196
Galactose (milk sugar), 199
Gall bladder, 115
    BMI as factor for gallstones, 169
Gangrene, 392
Gaseous exchange, 309
Gastric juices, 114

Gastrocnemius, 8f, 9f
  ankles, 30c
  calves, 28c
  synovial joint motions, 28c
Gastroesophageal reflux (GER), 129
Gastroesophageal reflux disease (GERD), 129
  complications related to, 130
Gastrointestinal (GI) tract, 107–109, 108f
  lower GI tract, 109
  upper GI tract, 107–108
Gender differences. See Male vs. female
Genetics
  aneurysm, 295
  coenzyme Q10 (CoQ10) effect on genetic disorders, 229
  Crohn's disease, risk of, 127
  dwarfism, 357
  muscle development, 203
  muscle fiber distribution, 11
  weight loss determined by, 183
GER (gastroesophageal reflux), 129
GERD (gastroesophageal reflux disease), 129, 130
Ghost image, 364
Gigantism, 415
GI tract. See Gastrointestinal (GI) tract
Glands, 377, 379–381
  adrenal glands, 380
  ceruminous glands, 384
  ear glands, 380, 384
  endocrine glands, 379–380
  exocrine glands, 379–380
  hypothalmus, 380
  lacrimal (tear) glands, 379, 380
  mammary glands, 379, 380, 383
  mucous glands, 380
  ovaries, 380
  pancreas, 380
  parathyroid, 380
  pineal, 380
  pituitary gland, 155, 330f, 380
  salivary glands, 113, 114, 379, 380
  sebaceous glands, 376f, 380, 391, 392
  sex glands, 391
  sudoriferous glands, 382, 383
  sweat glands, 379, 380, 382
  testes, 380
  thyroid, 380
Glare, 364
Glial cells, 333–335
Gliding (planar) joint, 91c
Glossary, 425–429
Glucagon, 155
Glucose (blood sugar), 114, 115, 161, 165–167. See also Insulin
  glycogen converted into, 201. See also Glycogens
  simple carbohydrates, 201
  simple sugar, 199, 201
Glutamic acid, 206
Glutamine, 206
Gluteus maximus, 9f, 31c
  synovial joint motions, 27c
Gluteus medius, 8f, 31c
  synovial joint motions, 27c
Gluteus minimus, 31c
  synovial joint motions, 27c
Glycemic index, 202

Glycine, 206
Glycogens, 167
    digestion of, 114
    ketosis, effect of, 145
    polysaccharides, 200
    production of, 167
    storage of, 115, 202
Golfers experiencing tennis elbow, 58
Gonadal hormones, 391
Gonads, 391
Goniometer test, 69
"Good" cholesterol. See HDL
Gout, 98
Gracilis, 8f, 9f
    knees, 30c
    synovial joint motions, 27c
Grains, 201, 216, 223, 230
Grand mal seizure, 354
    aura, 354
    clonic phase, 354
    postictal phase, 354
    tonic phase, 354
Great saphenous vein, 258f
Great vessels of the heart, 237f, 239
Grinding/crackling sound (crepitus)
    arthritis, 95
    cartilage (meniscus) tear, 64
    defined, 426
Groin, inguinal hernia in, 119
Growth
    abnormalities. See Body types and growth abnormalities
    endocrine system's role, 381
Gymnasts engaging in compulsive exercising, 144

H

Hair, 385–386
    alpecia (baldness), 403
    angora, 385
    dandruff, 392, 403
    definitive, 385
    functions of, 386
    lanugo, 385
    types of, 385
Hair bulb, 376f
Hair follicles, 376f, 377
Hair shaft, 376f
Hallucinations, seizures causing, 353
Halos, 364
Hammer (ear), 81
Hamstrings
    active stretching, 45
    dynamic (ballistic) stretching, 46
    primary joint motions, 30c
    reciprocal innervation inhibition as safeguard for, 50
    skeletal muscles, 30c
    workout chart, 180c
Hand-foot syndrome, 222
Hands. See also Carpals
    dorsal, 417
    finger nails, 387
    left-hand control, 332f
    palmer, 417
    rheumatoid arthritis, 97
    right-hand control, 332f
    synovial joint motions, 91c
Haze, 364
HDL (high-density lipoprotein) cholesterol, 210, 214, 290

    effects of eating on, 293
    hypercholesterolemia, 288
    range references, 292c
Head. *See also* Brain
    cephalo-, 417
    cranium bones, 78, 80
    injuries and conditions
        concussion, 57
        seizures as result of, 353
    joints, 85
    skull bones, 80–81
    sweat glands in forehead, 382
    temporal pulse site, 248
Headaches
    concussion, 57
    in grand mal seizure, 354
    hypoglycemia, 166
    hyponatremia, 187
    shingles (herpes zoster), 393
    stroke symptom, 296
Hearing, 331
Heart
    adrenaline's effect on, 163
    aorta, 237f, 239, 242f
    apex of, 248
    atrioventricular (mitral) valve, 242f
    atrioventricular (tricuspid) valve, 242f
    brachiocephalic artery, 242f
    brain functioning dependent on, 331
    cardio-, 417
    chambers, 241, 243
    circulation of blood through, 243–244
    diagram, 242f
    coenzyme Q10 (CoQ10) in, 229
    definition of, 235, 238
    diagram of, 237f
    ejection fraction, 250
    endocardium, 240
    epicardium, 240
    function of, 235, 238
    great vessels, 237f, 239
    healthy exercise for, 259–281. *See also* Exercise
    heart map, 243–244
    heart muscle. *See* Cardiac muscle
    hyperthyroidism's effect on, 157
    inferior vena cava, 237f, 239, 242f, 256, 258f
    interaction with lungs, 243–244
    layers of heart wall, 240
    left atrium, 237f, 241, 242f
    left common carotid artery, 242f
    left pulmonary arteries, 237f, 242f, 256
    left subclavian artery, 242f
    left ventricle, 237f, 241, 242f
    location in circulatory system, 258f
    lower chambers, 241
    measurements, 249–250. *See also* Heart rate
    mediastinum, 239
    myocardium, 240
    oxygen extraction, 250, 263
    pericardium, 237f, 239
    potassium's role, 227
    pulmonary arteries, 237f, 239, 242f
    pulmonary veins, 237f, 239

left pulmonary veins, 237f
right pulmonary veins, 237f, 242f
right atrium, 237f, 241, 242f
right pulmonary artery, 237f, 242f
right ventricle, 237f, 241, 242f, 256
septum, 242f
stroke volume, 250
structure of, 237f, 239
superior vena cava, 237f, 239, 242f, 256, 258f
upper chambers, 241
ventricles, 237f, 241, 242f, 250
visceral fat surrounding, 137
vitamin B-1 helping with, 221
Heart arrhythmias. See Cardiac arrhythmias
Heart attack. See Cardiac arrest; Myocardial infarction
Heart beat. See also Heart rate
beats per minute (bpm), 249
listening to, 245
Heartburn, 129
Heart chambers, 241, 243
Heart disease and conditions. See also Cardiac arrest; Myocardial infarction
angina (angina pectoris), 286
aortic stenosis, 286
arrhythmia. See Cardiac arrhythmias
arteriosclerosis (thickening/hardening of arteries), 286
atherosclerosis (thickening/hardening of arteries), 286, 287
BMI as factor for, 169

bradycardia, 285
coenzyme Q10's (CoQ10) benefits for, 229
coronary artery disease (CAD), 287
emphysema leading to, 318
free radicals causing, 228
ischemia, 286
myocarditis, 287
stroke, increasing risk with, 296
tachycardia, 286
vitamin B-9 deficiency causing, 223
wheezing associated with, 318
Heart healthy exercise, 259–281
beginner aerobic training guidelines, 264–270. See also Aerobic exercises
Borg Scale, 272
capacity to consume oxygen, 263
cardio endurance, 262
ergometer, 261
Karvonen Formula (also known as Heart Rate Maximum Reserve Method), 275–279
Max Cardiac Output, 263
maximum heart rate and calculations, 273–274
Max Oxygen Extraction, 263
MET system, 271
safe training, 280–281
stress tests. See Stress tests
talk test, 272
training heart rate range (THRR), 273
VO2 Max, 263
Heart map, 243–244
Heart muscle. See Cardiac muscle

Heart rate (HR), 249–250
    aerobic exercises' intensity, 264, 277
    arrhythmia. *See* Cardiac arrhythmias
    autonomic nervous system controlling, 328
    beats per minute (bpm), 249
    bradycardia, 285
    cardiac output, 249
    ejection fraction, 250
    ergometer to measure, 261
    Karvonen Formula (also known as Heart Rate Maximum Reserve Method), 275–279
    maximum. *See* Maximum heart rate (MHR)
    oxygen extraction, 250
    resting heart rate (RHR), 249, 251, 276–277
    stroke volume, 250
    tachycardia, 286
    training chart, 265*c*
Heat conditions, 185–187
    cramps, 186
    dehydration, 186. *See also* Dehydration
    heat exhaustion, 186
    heat stroke, 186
    hypernatremia, 187
    hypochloremia, 186
    hyponatremia, 187
Height. *See also* Dwarfism
    basal metabolic rate (BMR) factor, 159
Helicobacter pylori, 121
Hemarthrosis, 397
Hematoma, 397
Hemo- (body part designation), 417
Hemoglobin, 251, 288, 312
Hemorrhage, 397
Hemorrhoids, 124–125
Hernia, 119–120
    femoral, 120
    hiatal, 120
    inguinal, 119
    umbilical, 120
Herniated disk, 356
Herpes, 400
Herpes zoster. *See* Shingles
Hiatal hernia, 120
High blood-potassium level (hyperkalemia), 156
High blood pressure (hypertension), 155, 247
    BMI as factor, 169
    essential hypertension, 247
    stroke, increasing risk with, 296
    white coat hypertension, 247
High blood-sodium level (hypernatremia), 187
High-density lipoprotein cholesterol. *See* HDL
High-fructose corn syrup, 201
High jumping causing patellar tendonitis (jumpers knee), 63
Hinge joint, 91*c*
Hips, 79
    abduction, 27*c*, 31*c*
    adduction, 27*c*
    bones, 79
    circumduction motion, 90
    extension, 27*c*, 31*c*

fat cells, 138
flexion, 27c
injuries and conditions
    ankylosing spondylitis, 97
    bursitis, 56
    lateral rotation, 27c
    medial rotation, 27c
    synovial joint motions, 25, 27c, 91c
Histidine, 206
Hives (urticaria), 393
Hodgkin lymphoma, 409c, 413
Holding your breath while exercising, 319
Holistic thought, 332f
Homeostatis, 154, 155, 375
Honey, 201
Horizontal extension, 89
Horizontal flexion, 89
Hormones
    definition of, 381
    endocrine system's role, 381
    glands' role with, 379
    insulin. See Insulin
    pituitary hormones, 155
    plasma's role with, 252
    renin-angiotensin system, 155
    steriod hormones, 289
    thyroid, 157, 226
Humerus, 77f, 79, 89
Humming sound, 402
Hunger, endocrine system's role in feelings of, 381
Hyaline cartilage, 37
Hydrochloric acid, 225
Hydrogen, 207, 209, 210

Hydrogenation, 209, 214
Hydrolysis, 162, 426
Hyoid bone, 78
Hypercholesterolemia, 288
Hyperextension, 56, 100
Hyperkalemia (high blood-potassium level), 156
Hypernatremia (high blood-sodium level), 187
Hyperopia, 363
Hyperplasia, 18
Hypertension. See High blood pressure
Hyperthyroidism, 157
Hypertrophic scar tissue, 401
Hypertrophy, 17
Hyperventilation, 319
Hypodermis (subcutaneous), 376f, 377
Hypoglycemia, 164, 166
Hypokalemia, 156
Hypokinesis, 426
Hypotension, 187
Hypothalamus, 155
Hypothalmus, 330f
Hypothyroidism, 157

I

IBS (irritable bowel syndrome), 122–123
IBS-M (mixed IBS), 122
Ibuprofen, peptic ulcer caused by, 121
Ice cream, 201. See also Dairy products
Ice to relieve pain, 57, 58, 66
Ileum, 108f, 109, 111, 112
Iliac artery, 258f
Iliac vein, 258f

Ilio- (body part designation), 419
Iliopsoas, 27c
Iliotibial band (ITB), 64, 426
Iliotibial band syndrome, 64
Ilium, 77f
Imagination, 332f
Immune system
    cancers starting in, 409c, 410
    vitamin E boosting, 224
    zinc boosting, 227
Impetigo, 400
Improvement conditioning stage, 267
Incision, 396
Inclinometer test, 69
Incontinence, lumbar radiculopathy causing, 361
Indirect inguinal hernia, 119
Indolent cancer, 413
Infants. See also Congenital conditions
    brown fat cells of, 138
Infections
    seizures caused by, 353
    selenium's protective role, 227
    Vitamin A's protective role, 220
    Vitamin B-6's protective role, 222
    zinc's protective role, 227
Infective arthritis, 98
Inferior lobe, 303f, 308
Inferior nasal concha bones, 81
Inferior position, 418
Inferior rectus muscle, 344f
Inferior vena cava, 237f, 239, 242f, 256, 258f
Inflammation (as symptom), 398
    arthritis, 97

bronchitis, 317
bursitis, 56
cortisone to reduce, 101
Crohn's disease causing IBD, 126–128
gout, 98
ice to reduce, 66
iliotibial band syndrome (ITB), 64
jumpers knee, 63
myocarditis, 287
plantar fasciitis, 62
rheumatoid arthritis, 97, 358
shingles, 393
shoulder impingement, 58
skin, 391–392
spinal stenosis, 356
synovitis, 358
tendonitis, 56
tennis elbow, 58
tumors, 358
Inflammatory bowel disease
    Crohn's disease as, 126
    microscopic colitis, 126
    ulcerative colitis, 126
Infra- (position), 418
Infraspinatus, 33c
    synovial joint motions, 26c
Inguinal hernia, 119
Inhalation, 312
Initial conditioning stage, 267
Injuries and conditions
    brain. See Brain
    cartilage. See Cartilage
    circulatory system. See Circulatory system injuries and conditions

digestive system. *See* Digestive system injuries and conditions
integumentary system. *See* Integumentary system injuries and conditions
joints. *See* Joints
knees. *See* Knees
legs. *See* Legs
muscular system. *See* Muscular system injuries and conditions
nervous system. *See* Nervous system injuries and conditions
patella. *See* Patella
respiratory system. *See* Respiratory system injuries and conditions
rotator cuffs. *See* Rotator cuffs
shoulders. *See* Shoulders
skeletal. *See* Skeletal injuries and conditions
spinal cord. *See* Nervous system injuries and conditions
spine. *See* Spine
tendon. *See* Tendon; Tendonitis
Insertion
   bone that moves, 419
   distal bone, 419
   tendon insertion, 21
Insight, 332*f*
Institute of Medicine recommended daily intakes of omega-6 fatty acid, 212
Insulin, 115, 155, 164, 165
   chromium's role with, 226
Integumentary system, 371–387. *See also* Skin
   endocrine glands, 379–380
   endocrine system, 381
   epithelial tissues, 379
   exocrine glands, 379–380
   glands, 379–381. *See also* Glands
   hair, 385–386
   injuries and conditions. *See* Integumentary system injuries and conditions
   nails, 387
   skin layers, 376. *See also* Skin
      diagram of, 376*f*
Integumentary system injuries and conditions, 389–404
   bleeding, 397
   contusion (bruise), 397
   ecchymosis, 397
   hemarthrosis, 397
   hematoma, 397
   hemorrhage, 397
   symptoms, 398–399
      edema, 399
      effusion, 399
      inflammation, 398
      swelling, 398
Intercostal muscles, 311, 312
Intermediate slow distance, 268
Internal hemorrhoids, 124
Internal oblique, 31*c*
   workout chart, 180*c*
Internal respiration, 302
Internal rotators, 27*c*
Interval training, 269
Intervertebral disks. *See* Disks
Intervertebral foramen (neural foramen), 340
Intestines. *See also* Large intestine; Small intestine

Crohn's disease and, 126–127
visceral muscle in, 7
Intraocular pressure (IOP), 349
tonometry to determine, 365
Intuition, 332f
Inversion of foot, 30c, 90
Involuntary actions, 325
medulla controlling, 331
Involuntary muscles. See Muscular system
Involuntary nervous system. See Autonomic nervous system
Iodine, 218, 219, 226
IOP (intraocular pressure), 349
tonometry to determine, 365
Iris, 344, 344f, 378
Iron, 218, 226
Irritability caused by hypoglycemia, 166
Irritable bowel syndrome (IBS), 122–123
Ischium, 77f
Islets (or Islands) of Langerhans, 115, 164, 426
Isoleucine, 206
Isometric contractions, 19, 47
ITB (iliotibial band), 64, 426
Itching, 392, 393
IU (international units), 196

J

Jugular vein, 258f
Jaw. See also Teeth
bone (mandible), 77f, 81
salivary glands in, 114
Jejunum, 109, 110
Joint cavity, 84
Joints, 84
also called articulations, 84, 419
arthritis. See Arthritis
arthro- (body part designation), 419
cartilaginous joints (synchondroses), 85
defined, 84
facet joints, 340
fibrous joints (syndesmoses), 85
flexibility of, 42
injuries and conditions
arthralgia, 425
dislocation, 56
hemarthrosis, 397
hyperextension, 56
sprains of joint capsules, 55
subluxation, 56
muscle stabilization of, 21
nutrition of, 37, 84
synovial. See Synovial joints
types of, 85
Jumpers knee (patellar tendonitis), 63

K

Karvonen Formula (also known as Heart Rate Maximum Reserve Method), 275–279
Keloid scar tissue, 401
Keratectomy, 368
Keratin, 378
Keratitis, 364
Keratoconus, 362
Keratomileusis, 368
Keratotomy, 368
Ketosis, 145
Kidney failure

bulimia causing, 146
diabetes causing, 165
hyperkalemia caused by, 156
hyperventilation caused by, 319
hypokalemia caused by, 156
Kidneys
    blood pressure regulation, 155
    coenzyme Q10 (CoQ10) in, 229
    location in circulatory system, 258f
    potassium's role, 227
    protein consumption, danger of excessive, 204
Kilocalorie, 191
Knees
    extension, 28c, 30c
    flexion, 28c, 30c
    gracilis, 30c
    iliotibial band (ITB), 64, 426
    injuries and conditions
        ankylosing spondylitis, 97
        anterior cruciate ligament (ACL) tears, 64
        bursitis, 56
        chondromalacia patella, 62, 63
        iliotibial band syndrome (ITB), 64
        patellar tendonitis (jumpers knee), 63
        patellofemoral pain syndrome, 63
        torn meniscus (cartilage), 37, 64
    meniscus, 37, 64
    primary joint motions, 30c
    semitendinosus, 30c
    skeletal muscles, 30c
    synovial joint motions, 25, 28c, 91c
    synovial joints, 85
Korotkoff sounds, 246
Kyphosis, 100

L

LA (linoleic acid), 212
Laceration, 396
Lacrimal bones, 81
Lacrimal gland, 346
Lactate (lactic acid), 164, 427
Lacto-ovo vegetarians, 428
Lactose (milk sugar), 199, 201
Lacto vegetarians, 428
Lamina, 340
Language ability, 332f
Lanugo (hair on fetus), 385
Lard, 209
Large blisters (bullae), 400
Large calorie, 191
Large intestine, 108f, 109, 112
    Crohn's disease and, 126
Larynx (voice box), 303f, 304, 305
Laser, 368
Laser keratome, 367
LASIK, 368
Lateral plane. See Sagittal plane
Lateral position, 418
Lateral rotation
    abdominals, 31c
    arm, 33c
    hip, 27c
    shoulder, 26c, 33c
Latissimus dorsi, 8f, 9f, 21, 32c
    synovial joint motions, 26c
    workout chart, 180c

Laxatives, 146
LDL (low-density lipoprotein) cholesterol, 209, 210, 212, 214, 291
    effects of eating on, 293
    hypercholesterolemia, 288
    range references, 292c
Lean body mass, 136, 137
    determining, 149
    muscle size's effect on, 149
Learning disabilities, 325
Left atrium, 237f, 241, 242f
Left brain functions, 332f
Left common carotid artery, 242f
Left-hand control, 332f
Left lung, 309
Left pulmonary arteries, 237f, 242f, 256
Left pulmonary veins, 237f, 242f
Left subclavian artery, 242f
Left ventricle, 237f, 241, 242f
Legal blindness, 363
Leg curls, 21
    workout chart, 180c
Leg extensions, 21, 22
    dynamometer test during, 68
    patellofemoral pain syndrome from, 63
    workout chart, 180c
Leg press
    benefits of, 178
    workout chart, 180c
Legs. See also Ankles; Calves; Feet; Hamstrings; Knees; Quadriceps
    concentric contractions, 30c
    injuries and conditions, 60–64
        Achilles tendonitis and rupture, 62
        ankle sprains, 61
        anterior cruciate ligament (ACL) tears, 64
        biomechanical problems, 63
        cartilage (meniscus) tear, 37, 64
        chondromalacia patella, 62, 63
        iliotibial band syndrome (ITB), 64
        muscle imbalances, 63
        patellar tendonitis (jumpers knee), 63
        patellofemoral pain syndrome, 63
        plantar fasciitis, 62
        shin splints, 61
    lumbar radiculopathy causing pain in, 361
    muscle groups, 30c
    numbness, 356
    primary joint motions, 30c
    skeletal muscles, 30c
    workout chart, 180c
Legumes, 201
Lens, 344, 344f
Leucine, 206
Leukemia, 220, 409c, 410, 413
Leukocytes. See White blood cells
Lifestyle, effects of, 136
Lifting. See also Body building
    biceps curl, 19
    hemorrhoids, causes of, 124
    motor units, 23
Ligamen anteriosum, 237f
Ligaments, 36, 84, 340
    defined, 84
    normal joint vs. osteoarthritis, 96f

sprains, 55
Ligamentum flavum, 340
Lightheadedness
　heat exhaustion, 186
　hypoglycemia, 166
　warm-up and cool-down preventing, 181–182, 270
Linoleic acid (LA), 212
Lipids, 208, 213, 289, 291. See also Cholesterol; Triglycerides
　free radicals damaging, 228
Lipoproteins, 289–290, 293
Lips, discoloration of, 318
Liver, 115
　both exocrine and endocrine glands, 381
　cholesterol produced by, 289, 290
　coenzyme Q10 (CoQ10) in, 229
　storage of glycogen in, 115, 202
　visceral fat surrounding, 137
LNA (alpha-linolenic acid), 212
Lobes, 304, 308, 309
Lobular carcinoma, 409c, 411
Logic, 332f
Long slow distance, 268
Lordosis, 100
Loss of consciousness. See also Fainting or feeling faint; Unconsciousness
　brain's lack of oxygen causing, 331
　in grand mal seizure, 354
　heat stroke, 186
　hypoglycemia, 166
　seizures causing, 353
Loss of speech. See Speech, loss of or difficulties with

Low blood-potassium level (hypokalemia), 156
Low blood pressure, 155
Low blood-sodium level (hyponatremia), 187
Low-density lipoprotein cholesterol. See LDL
Lower back
　ankylosing spondylitis, 97
　lumbar vertebrae, 82f, 83, 419
　pain, 57
Lower GI tract, 109
Lower heart chambers, 241
Lowering motion in biceps curls, 19
Lower respiratory tract, 304, 307–309
Lower trapezius, 32c
Low vision, 363
Luekocytes, 427
Lumbar (body part designation), 417
Lumbar radiculopathy, 361
Lumbar vertebrae, 82f, 83, 419
Lung cancer, 422
Lungs, 235, 242f, 304, 309, 311
Lycopene, 228
Lymphoma, 409c, 410, 411, 413
Lymph vessels, 377
Lysine, 206

M
Macro minerals, 219
Macrosomia, 415
Macula, 345
Magnesium, 218, 219, 225, 226
Maintenance conditioning stage, 268, 270

Male vs. female
    basal metabolic rate (BMR), 159
    body composition, 136
    body fat percentages, 173
    breast cancer, 411
    cellulite, 137
    direct inguinal hernia, 119
    facial hair growth, 385
    femoral hernia, 120
    to lose one to two pounds per week, 141
    muscular structure, 11, 17
Malignancy, 409c, 410, 411
Malnutrition
    compulsive exercising, 144
    Crohn's disease and, 127
Maltose, 114, 199, 201
Malt sugar. *See* Maltose
Mandible (jaw bone), 77f, 81
Manganese, 218, 226
Margarine, 209, 214
Max Cardiac Output, 263
Maxilla bones, 81
Maximum heart rate (MHR), 265c
    calculations, 273–274
        for lower and upper limits, 274
    compared to aerobic capacity, 275
    formula, 273
    safe training guidelines, 280
Max Oxygen Extraction, 263
mcg (µg) (micrograms), 196
Meals. *See* Diet
Meat consumption, 213, 216
    cholesterol levels, 289, 294
    vitamin B-1 from, 221
    vitamin B-2 from, 221
    vitamin B-6 from, 222
Medial position, 418
Medial rotation
    arm, 33c
    hip, 27c
    leg (tibia), 30c
    pectoralis major, 33c
    shoulder, 26c
Mediastinum, 239, 309
Medical terminology, 421–422
    acute condition or symptom, 422
    chronic condition or symptom, 422
    diagnosis, 421
    idiopathic conditions, 422
    primary risk factor, 422
    prognosis, 421
    risk factor, 422
    stenosis, 422
Medulla, 330f, 331, 378
Melanin, 378
Melanoma (skin cancer), 392, 409c, 412
Melatonin, 380
Membranes, 337
Memory, 331
Memory difficulties, 57, 325
Menaquinone-4, 224
Menaquinone-7 (vitamin K2), 224
Meniscus, 37. *See also* Torn mensicus or cartilage
Menstrual cycle
    amenorrhea (absence of monthly periods), 143
    bulimia's effect on, 146
    hyperthyroidism's effect on, 157

Men vs. women. *See* Male vs. female
Mesomorph, 416
Metabolism, 142, 158. *See also* Basal metabolic rate (BMR)
    compulsive exercising and metabolic disorders, 144
    muscle tissue burning calories and, 150
    set-point theory and, 152
    starvation and, 145
    thyroid hormones' role, 226
Metacarpals, 77f, 79
Metatarsals, 77f, 79
Methionine, 206
MET system, 271
mg (milligrams), 196
Microkeratome, 368
Microscopic colitis, 126
Midbrain, 330f
Middle deltoids, 26c, 33c
Middle lobe, 303f, 308
Middle trapezius, 32c
Milk, 201, 209, 221, 222. *See also* Dairy products
Milk sugar, 199
Minerals, 193, 195
    descriptions of, 225–227
    essential minerals, 218
    macro minerals, 219
    trace minerals, 219
Mitochondria, 12f, 13
Mitosis, 334
Mixed IBS (IBS-M), 122
Molasses, 201
Mole (skin), 393

Molybdenum, 218, 227
Monosaccharides, 199
Monounsaturated fatty acids, 210
Monovision, 368
Motor commands, 24
Motor learning factor, 24
Motor neurons, 24
Motor units, 23
Mouth, 107, 113, 304, 305, 312. *See also* Teeth
    salivary glands, location in, 114
    sores from deficient B-2 intake, 221
    sores from deficient B-6 intake, 222
Mucous colitis, 122
Mucus, 305, 306, 317
Multiplanar plane, motion on, 90
Multiple myeloma, 409c, 410
Multiple sclerosis, 335
Muscle coordination, 331
Muscle fatigue, 164
Muscle fiber. *See* Muscular system
Muscle spindle activity, 46, 48
Muscle weakness
    coenzyme Q10 (CoQ10) effects, 229
    hyperkalemia symptom, 156
    hyponatremia, 187
    radiculopathy, 357, 360
Muscular dystrophy, 68
Muscular system
    adrenaline's effect on, 163
    agonist muscle, 21–22, 41, 45, 46, 50
    antagonist muscle, 21–22, 41, 45, 46, 50

basal metabolic rate (BMR) as factor in maintaining muscle mass, 159
best age for strength gain, 17
BMI overestimating body fat for those with muscular build, 169
building muscles. See Body building
calorie burning by adding muscle, 147–148, 150–151, 158
cardiac muscle, 6f, 7
    muscle force, 18
    sarcolemma, 12f, 13
characteristics of muscles, 16–22
    agonist muscle, 21–22
    antagonist muscle, 21–22
    atrophy, 18
    contractions. See below: contractions
    hyperplasia, 18
    hypertrophy, 17
    muscle attachment relating to a limb, 20
    muscle attachment relating to a motion, 20
    muscle force, 18, 23
    muscle pairs, 41, 45, 46
    muscle size, 17–18
    quadriceps, 22
    stabilization, 21
    synergist muscle, 22
    tendon insertion, 21. See also Tendon
components of muscle, 5
conditions. See Muscular system injuries and conditions
connective tissue types, 36–37. See also Tendon
    cartilage, 37
    fascia, 36
    ligaments, 36
contractions
    agonist muscle, 21–22, 41, 45, 46, 50
    antagonist muscle, 21–22, 41, 45, 46, 50
    ATP's role, 167
    calcium's role in, 225
    Central Nervous System, 13
    compared to stretching and stabilization, 41
    concentric contractions, 19–20, 29
    description of, 18
    eccentric contractions, 19
    fast speed of, 10
    in grand mal seizure, 354
    interdependent skeletal muscle fibers, 15
    isometric contractions, 19, 47
    moving bone (insertion), 419
    muscle force, 18
    muscular reflex contraction, 46
    neuromuscular system, 23
    pulling, not pushing, by muscles, 20
    reciprocal innervation inhibition to safeguard against, 50
    safety responses to, 50–51
    sarcomeres, 13, 17

slow speed of, 11
sodium's role, 227
stationary bone (origin), 419
distal attachment, 20
function of, 5
genetics as factor for muscle development, 203
hyperthyroidism's effect on, 157
injuries. See Muscular system injuries and conditions
involuntary muscles
   cardiac muscle, 7
   smooth (visceral) muscles, 7
   tissues, 6f
lean body mass, effect of muscle size on, 149
lengthening muscle, 19, 41
loss of muscle as people age, 203
maintaining muscle tissue, 150
motor commands, 24
motor learning factor, 24
motor neurons, 24
motor units, 23
muscle attachment, 20
muscle fiber, 10–13
   also called muscle cells, 13
   composition and function, 12
   distribution of, 11
   increase in size (hypertrophy), 17
   mitochondria, 12f, 13
   muscle force related to size of, 18
   myofibrils, 12f, 13, 17
   nucleus, 12f, 13
   sarcolemma, 12f, 13
   sarcomeres, 13, 17

sliding filament theory, 13
muscle loss as people age, 203
muscle spindle activity, 46, 48
muscle tissue, 423
myo-, 417
nervous inhibition, 24
neuromuscular system, 23–24
number of muscles, 5
origin of muscle attachment, 20
overview, 5
protein and water composition of muscle tissue, 203
proximal attachment, 20
shortening muscle, 19, 29, 41
skeletal muscles, 6f, 7
   back view (diagram with names of muscles), 9f
   endoysium, 14f, 15
   epimysium tendons, 14f, 15
   fascicles, 14f, 15
   fast-twitch white muscle fiber, 10, 23
   front & side view (diagram with names of muscles), 8f
   functions of, 7
   interdependent skeletal muscle fibers, 15
   major muscles and their joint motions, 29
   muscle force, 18, 23
   perimysium, 14f, 15
   sarcolemma, 12f, 13
   slow-twitch red muscle fiber, 10, 11, 23
   structure of (diagram with names of structures), 14f

Type 1 muscle fiber, 11
Type 2 muscle fiber, 10
types of muscle fiber, 10
smooth muscle, 6f, 7
stabilization, 41
stabilizer muscles, 21
stretching, 41
    autogenic inhibition to safeguard against excessive stretching, 51
    compared to contraction and stabilization, 41
    contract/relax method, 47
    defined, 44
    dynamic (ballistic) stretches, 46, 48
    myotatic reflex, 48
    neurophysiological effects of, 48–49
    overstretching (stretch weakness), 65
    proprioceptive neuromuscular facilitation (PNF), 47
    proprioceptors, 49
    safety responses to, 50–51
    static stretch, 44
    types of, 44–47
synovial joint motions, 25, 26–28c
tendon. See Tendon
testing devices, 68–69
types of muscle tissue, 6
voluntary muscles, 5, 29
    skeletal muscle, 7
    tissues, 6f
water and protein composition of muscle tissue, 203
weight lifting, development of muscle tissue, 147
Muscular system injuries and conditions, 53–68
    biceps tendon rupture, 58
    bursitis, 56, 58
    common types of, 55–59
    concussion, 57
    dislocation, 56
    dynamometer test to detect, 68
    EMGs (electromyograms) to detect, 68
    fasting causing atrophy, 144
    goniometer test to detect, 69
    hematoma, 397
    hyperextension, 56
    inclinometer test to detect, 69
    leg injuries and conditions, 60–64. See also Legs
    low back pain, 57
    overstretching (stretch weakness), 65
    peripheral nerve damage, 68
    pinching injury, 58
    RICE technique to treat, 61, 63, 66–67
    rotator cuff tear, 59
    shoulder impingement syndrome, 58
    sprains vs. strains, 55
    subluxation, 56
    tendonitis, 56
    tennis elbow (epicondylitis), 58
    testing devices, 68–69
    torn meniscus, 37, 64
Music awareness, 332f

Myasthenia gravis, 68
Mydriatic drops to dilate eyes, 365
Myelin, 333f, 335
Myelin sheath, 335
Myo- (body part designation), 417
Myocardial infarction, 287. See also
    Cardiac arrest
    fish oil's omega-3 fatty acids protecting against, 212
    HDL protecting against, 290
    trans fatty acids increasing risk of, 214
    triglycerides increasing risk of, 213
Myocardium, 240
Myocytes, 240, 427
Myofibrils, 12f, 13, 14f, 17
Myoglobin, 427
Myopia, 363
Myosin, 13, 17
Myotatic reflex, 48
    Golgi tendon organ, 48, 51
    muscle spindles, 48, 50

N

Nail polish, 387
Nails, 387
Nasal bones, 81
Nasal cavity, 303f
Nausea from heat exhaustion, 186
Nearsightedness, 363
Neck. See also Cervical vertebrae
    carotid pulse site, 248
    cervical, 417
    hyperextension, 100
    muscles, 311
    synovial joint motions, 91c
Necrosis of body tissue, 392
Neoplasm, 409c, 411
Nerve endings, 376f, 377
Nerves. See also Neurons
    calcium's role, 225
    components of, 333
    magnesium's role, 226
    motor neurons, 24
    nerve tissue, 423
    neuroglia (glial cells), 333–335
    peripheral nerve damage, 68
    sodium's role, 227
    vitamin B-1 helping with, 221
    vitamin B-6 helping with, 222
    vitamin B-12 helping with, 223
Nervous colon, 122
Nervous inhibition, 24
Nervous system, 321–350. See also Brain; Neurons; Spinal cord
    autonomic nervous system, 328
    central nervous system, 325, 327
    division of, 325
    parasympathetic nervous system, 329
    peripheral nervous system, 325, 328–329
    potassium's role, 227
    sympathetic nervous system, 329
Nervous system injuries and conditions, 351–369
    achondroplasia, 357
    acquired causes, 359–361
        ossification of the posterior longitudinal ligament, 360

Paget's disease, 360
  radiculopathy, 360–361
  trauma, 359
  tumors of the spine, 359
 arthritis types, 358
  rheumatoid arthritis, 358
  spondylosis, 358
  synovitis, 358
 brain. See Brain
 causes of, 325
 epilepsy, 354
 grand mal seizure, 354
  aura, 354
  clonic phase, 354
  postictal phase, 354
  tonic phase, 354
 herniated disk, 356
 radiculopathy, 357
 sciatica, 356, 357
 seizures (convulsions), 353–354. See also Seizures
 spinal stenosis, 356, 358, 359–360
 spondylolisthesis, 357
 types of, 327
 vitamin B-6 deficiency as cause, 222
 vitamin B-7 protecting against, 222
Neuroblastoma, 409c, 411
Neuroendocrine carcinoma, 409c, 412
Neuroglia (glial cells), 333–335
 oligodendrocytes, 335
Neuromuscular system, 23–24
Neurons, 334
 amitotic, 334
 axons, 333f, 334
  demyelination of, 335
  unmyelinated and myelinated, 335
 components of, 334
 dendrites, 333f, 334
 function of, 333, 334
 glial cells, 333–335
 melanin of pigment-bearing neurons, 378
 motor neurons, 24
 myelin, 333f, 335
 myelin sheath, 335
 nodes of Ranvier, 333f, 335
 nucleus, 333f
 soma, 333f, 334
 structure of, 333f
Nevus (mole or birthmark), 393
Niacin (vitamin B-3), 217, 218, 221
Nicotinic acid. See Vitamin B-3
Nodes of Ranvier, 333f, 335
Nonessential amino acids, 205–206
Non-Hodgkin lymphoma, 409c, 413
Nonsteroidal anti-inflammatory drugs (NSAIDs), 121
Nose, 304, 305, 312
 nasal bones, 81
 rhinoplasty (cosmetic surgery), 404
Nose hairs, 306
NSAIDs (nonsteroidal anti-inflammatory drugs), 121
Nucleus, 333f
 defined, 427
 muscle fiber, 12f, 13, 14f
Numbers, anatomical, 420
Number skills, 332f
Numbness

hand-foot syndrome, 222
hyperventilation, 319
radiculopathy, 357, 360
spinal stenosis, 356
Nutrient density, 194
Nutrition and nutrients. See Diet
Nuts, 201, 212, 222, 224, 230

O

Oats, 201
Obesity
    body fat percentages, 173
    body mass index (BMI), 169, 172c
    femoral hernia and, 120
    gastroesophageal reflux disease (GERD) and, 129
Occipital bone, 80
Oligodendrocytes, 335
Olive oil, 210
Omega-3 polyunsaturated fatty acids, 210, 211–212
Omega-6 polyunsaturated fatty acids, 210, 211–212
Opposition, 90
Optic cup, 347
Optic disc (optic nerve head), 347
Optic nerve, 342, 344f, 345
Oral cavity, 303f
Origin (stationary bone), 419
Origin attachment, 20
Ossification, 427
Ossification of the posterior longitudinal ligament, 360
Oste- (bone descriptor), 419
Osteoarthritis, 64, 96f, 97, 358

Osteophytes, 97
Osteoporosis, 188
Overcorrection, 368
Overfat as preferred term, 172
Overstretching (stretch weakness), 65
Overweight, 172. See also Obesity
    body mass index (BMI), 172c
Ovo vegetarians, 428
Oxidation, 228
Oxygen, 228, 235, 250, 253
    body's need for, 301
    brain's need for, 331
    capacity to consume oxygen, 263
    functional oxygen capacity (VO2 max), 271
    maximum oxygen consumption, 271
    Max Oxygen Extraction, 263
    respiration, 302, 309
Oxygen extraction, 250
    Max Oxygen Extraction, 263
Oxygen free radicals. See Free radicals

P

Paget's disease, 360
Pain relief
    cortisone injections, 56, 62, 63, 101
    ice, use of, 57, 58, 66
    RICE (rest, ice, compression, elevation) techniques, 66–67
Painters experiencing shoulder impingement syndrome, 58
Palatine bones, 81
Palmaris longus, 8f, 9f
Palmer (body part designation), 417

Palm oil, 209
Palms
    pronation motion, 90
    standard anatomical position, 76
    supination motion, 90
    sweat glands, 382
Palpation, 248
Pancreas, 115, 155, 164, 380. *See also* Insulin
    both exocrine and endocrine glands, 381
    coenzyme Q10 (CoQ10) in, 229
    Islets (or Islands) of Langerhans, 164, 426
    tumors, 121
Pancreatic juice, 115
Pantothenic acid (vitamin B-5), 217, 218, 222
Paper bag, breathing into, 319
Paralysis
    hyperkalemia symptom, 156
    hypokalemia symptom, 156
    lumbar radiculopathy causing, 361
Paranasal sinus, 305
Parasympathetic nervous system, 329
Parietal bones, 80
Parotid glands, 114
Partially hydrogenated fat, 214
Patella, 77*f*, 79
    injuries and conditions
        chondromalacia patella, 62
        patellar tendonitis (jumpers knee), 63
        patellofemoral pain syndrome, 63

Patellar tendonitis (jumpers knee), 63
Patellofemoral pain syndrome, 63
Peanut oil, 210
Pectineus, 8*f*
Pectoralis major, 8*f*, 21, 33*c*
    synovial joint motions, 26*c*
    workout chart, 180*c*
Pedicles, 340
Pellagra, 221
Pelvis, 79
Peptic ulcer, 121
Pericardium, 237*f*, 239
Perimysium, 14*f*, 15
Peripheral nervous system, 325, 328–329
    autonomic nervous system, 328
    conscious nervous system, 328
    divisions of, 328–329
    Schwann cells, 335
    unconscious nervous system, 328
Peripheral vision, 350
Peristalsis, 108
Peroneus longus and brevis, 8*f*
    ankles, 30*c*
    feet, 30*c*
    synovial joint motions, 28*c*
Peroneus tertius, 28*c*
Personal fitness trainers
    body composition, determination of, 136
    exercise program, consulting for design of, 140, 160, 281
    training heart rate range (THRR), determination of, 273
Perspiration. *See* Sweating

Pesco vegetarians, 428
Petineus, 27c
Phalanges, 77f, 79
Pharynx (throat), 107, 114, 303f, 304, 305
Phenylalanine, 206
Phosphagens, 162, 167
Phosphate molecules. See ATP (adenosine triphosphate); CP (creatine phosphate)
Phosphorus, 75, 218, 219, 224, 225, 227
Photoreceptors, 346
Photo-refractive keratectomy (PRK), 369
Phylloquinone, 217, 224
Physicians, consultation of
    back pain, 57
    for large blisters (bullae), 400
    medical terminology, 421–422
    osteoporosis as problem, 188
    prior to aerobic exercise program, 140, 267, 280
    prior to body building program, 140, 178
    prior to RICE technique use, 66
    prior to weight-loss program, 139–141, 216
    weight-loss problems and eating disorders, 143
    white coat hypertension caused by, 247
Phytochemicals (plant chemicals), 230
Phytonadione (vitamin K1), 224
Piles (hemorrhoids), 124
Pimples. See Acne; Skin conditions
Pinched nerves, 360–361

Pinching injury, 58
Pituitary gland, 155, 330f, 380, 415
Pivot (swivel) joint, 91c
Planar joint, 91c
Plantar (body part designation), 417
Plantar fasciitis, 62, 427
Plantar flexion, 30c, 90
Plantaris, 30c
Plant foods, 210, 216, 224, 294
Plasma, 251
Plastic elongation deformation, 43
Platelets (thrombocytes), 251, 252, 428
Pleura, 304, 308
Plyometrics, 46
Poison, 353
Polyps, 412
Polysaccharides, 200
Polyunsaturated fatty acids, 210
Pons, 330f
Popliteus, 30c
Posterior chamber, 347
Posterior (rear) deltoids, 26c, 33c
Posterior tibial arteries, 258f
Posterior tibialis, 28c
    ankles, 30c
    feet, 30c
Posterior tibial veins, 258f
Postules, 392
Posture
    anormalities, 100
    good posture, 416
    skeletal bones maintaining, 75
Potassium, 75, 218, 219, 227
    bulimia depleting, 146
    high blood-potassium level (hyperkalemia), 156

low blood-potassium level, 156
Pregnancy. *See also* Fetus
    femoral hernia and, 120
    gastroesophageal reflux disease (GERD) and, 129
    hemorrhoids, causes of, 124
    iodine importance during, 226
    zinc's role, 227
Presbyopia, 363
Primary risk factor, 422
PRK (photo-refractive keratectomy), 369
Processed foods, 213
Prognosis, 421
Proline, 206
Pronation of arm, 34c, 35c, 90
Pronator teres, 35c
Prone, 427
Proprioceptive neuromuscular facilitation (PNF), 47
Proprioceptors, 49
Prostate cancer, 409c, 411
Proteins, 139, 145, 152, 195
    athletes' daily requirements, 204
    calories per gram, 192
    cautions on consuming extra protein, 197, 204
    chromium's role with, 226
    free radicals damaging, 228
    muscle tissue, composition of, 203
    phosphorus's role with, 227
    suggested daily intakes, 197, 203
    supplements, 204
    zinc's role with, 227
Proximal attachment, 20
Proximal position, 418

origin (proximal bone), 419
Psoriasis, 97, 392, 403
Psychological functions
    nervous inhibition, 24
    nervous system impairment causing difficulty, 325
Ptyalin, 113, 114
Pubic area, sweat glands in, 382
Pull-down exercise
    safe method for, 56
    workout chart, 180c
Pulmonary arteries, 237f, 239, 255, 258f, 307, 310, 312
Pulmonary blood vessels, 310
Pulmonary edema, 319
Pulmonary veins, 237f, 239, 242f, 257, 258f, 307, 310
Pulse, 248, 256
Puncture, 396
Pupil (eye), 344, 344f
    autonomic nervous system controlling diameter of, 328
Pushing motion, 20
Push-ups, 20
Pyogenic conditions, 427
    infective arthritis, 98
Pyridoxine (vitamin B-6), 217, 218, 222
Pyruvate, 164, 427

Q

Quadriceps, 22
    concentric contractions of, 29, 30c
    passive stretching, 45
    primary joint motions, 30c
    reciprocal innervation inhibition as safeguard for, 50

workout chart, 180c
Quick reference
    anatomical positions, 418
    bone and cartilage terms, 419
    parts of body, 417
Quinoa, 201

R
Radial arteries, 248, 258f
Radial keratotomy (RK), 369
Radial pulse site, 248
Radiculopathy, 357, 360–361
    cervical radiculopathy, 361
    lumbar radiculopathy, 361
    thoracic radiculopathy, 361
Radius, 77f, 79, 85
    fibrous joints (syndesmoses), 85
Raising arms above head, pain caused by, 58
Range of motion, 428
    flexibility, 42
    goniometer test for, 69
    inclinometer test for, 69
Rear deltoids. See Posterior deltoids
Reasoning abilities, 331, 332f
Reciprocal innervation inhibition, 50
Rectum, 108f, 109, 112
    hemorrhoids, 124
Rectus abdominis, 8f, 31c
    workout chart, 180c
Rectus femoris, 8f, 22
    legs (quadriceps), 30c
    synovial joint motions, 27c, 28c
Red blood cells (erythrocytes), 75, 251, 253, 426

copper's role in formation of, 226
vitamins need for production of, 221–223
Redness
    arthritis, 95, 97
    burns, 395
    eczema, 392
    erythema, 391
    hand-foot syndrome, 222
    heat stroke, 186
    inflammation, 398
Reed-Sternberg cell, 413
Reflex actions. See also Coughing; Sneezing
    autonomic nervous system controlling, 328
Refraction, 365
Refractive errors, 364
Refractive power, 350
    refraction test for, 365
Relating to surroundings (proprioceptors), 49
Renal failure. See Kidney failure
Renal vein, 258f
Renin-angiotensin system, 155
Resistance to motion, 42
    resistance exercises, 184, 188, 203. See also Weight lifting
Resistive force, 19
Respiratory system, 297–313. See also Breathing
    abdominal muscles, 311
    airways, 304, 305
    alveolar ducts, 304, 307, 308
    alveolar sacs, 308

alveoli, 303f, 304, 307–309, 312, 317
autonomic nervous system controlling, 328
bronchial tree, 304, 308
bronchioles, 303f, 304, 307, 309
bronchus/bronchi, 303f, 304, 307–309
cellular respiration, 302
cilia, 304, 306
components of, 301
diagram of, 303f
diaphragm, 303f, 311–313
epiglottis (Adams apple), 303f, 304, 306
exhalation, 313
fissures, 304, 308
frontal sinus, 303f, 304, 305
functions of, 301
inferior lobe, 303f, 308
inhalation, 312
intercostal muscles, 311, 312
larynx (voice box), 303f, 304, 305
lobes, 304, 308, 309
lower respiratory tract, 304, 307–309
lungs, 304, 309, 311
mediastinum, 309
middle lobe, 303f, 308
mouth, 304, 305, 312. *See also* Mouth
muscles used for breathing, 311–313
nasal cavity, 303f
nose, 304, 305, 312
oral cavity, 303f
paranasal sinus, 305
pharynx (throat), 303f, 304, 305
pleura, 304, 308
pulmonary artery, 310, 312
pulmonary blood vessels, 310
pulmonary vein, 310
respiration, described, 302
sphenoid sinus, 303f, 304, 305
superior lobe, 303f, 308
trachea (windpipe), 303f, 304, 305, 307–309
upper respiratory tract, 304, 305–306
Respiratory system injuries and conditions, 315–319
aerophagia, 319
asthma, 318
bronchial asthma, 318
bronchitis, 317, 318
chronic obstructive pulmonary disease (COPD), 318
cyanosis, 318
dyspnea, 317
emphysema, 318
exercise-induced asthma, 318
gastroesophageal reflux disease (GERD) and, 130
hyperventilation, 319
suffocation, 317
valsalva maneuver, 319
Rest
basal metabolic rate (BMR) for, 7, 142, 159–160
burning calories while resting, 147, 150, 160

in fitness program, 140
parasympathetic nervous system controlling, 329
Rest, ice, compression, elevation (RICE techniques), 66–67
Resting heart rate (RHR), 249, 251, 276–277
Restive force, 428
Retina, 342, 344f, 345
Retinal pigment epithelium (RPE), 347
Retinoic acid, 220
Retinol (vitamin A), 217, 218, 220, 228
Rheumatoid arthritis, 97, 358
Rhomboids, 9f, 32c, 89
RHR (resting heart rate), 249, 251, 276–277
Riboflavin (vitamin B-2), 217, 218, 221
Ribs, 77f, 78
    cartilaginous joints (synchondroses), 85
    costo- (body part designation), 419
Rice, 201
RICE (rest, ice, compression, elevation) techniques, 66–67
Rickets, 224
Right atrium, 237f, 241, 242f
Right brain functions, 332f
Right-hand control, 332f
Right lung, 309
Right pulmonary artery, 237f, 242f
Right pulmonary veins, 237f, 242f
Right ventricle, 237f, 241, 242f, 256
Ringing sound, 402
Risk factor, 422
Risk factors for heart attack, 213, 214, 291
Risk factors for stroke, 213, 214, 291, 296
RK (radial keratotomy), 369
RNA, 13, 223, 427
Rods (rod cells), 347
Rotary motion, 89
Rotation, 89, 91c. *See also* Lateral rotation; Medial rotation
Rotator cuffs
    description of, 59
    injuries and conditions
        pinching injury (shoulder impingement), 58
        rotator cuff tear, 59
        rotator cuff tendinitis, 58
    primary joint motions, 33c
    skeletal muscles, 33c
Rowing machines, 261
    workout chart, 180c
RPE (retinal pigment epithelium), 347
Rubbing causing blisters, 394
Runners
    burning calories, 147
    compulsive exercising, 144
    dynamic (ballistic) stretches, 46
    endorphins produced by, 163
    injuries and conditions common to
        iliotibial band syndrome (ITB), 64
        patellofemoral pain syndrome, 63
        plantar fasciitis, 62
        shin splints, 61
        stress fracture, 99
        torn meniscus (cartilage), 64
    protein supplements, 204
    slow-twitch muscle fiber, 11

Rupture
    Achilles tendonitis and rupture, 62
    biceps tendon rupture, 58
    tendon, 56, 62, 63
Ruptured disks, 57

S

Sacrum, 82f, 83
Sacrum pubis, 77f
Saddle joint, 91c
Safflower oil, 210, 212
Sagittal (lateral) plane, 86, 87f
    motion on, 88, 90
Saliva, 113, 306, 328
Salivary glands, 113, 114, 379, 380
Salt. See Sodium
Saltatory conduction, 335
Salt tablets, 187
Sarcolemma, 12f, 13, 14f, 428
Sarcoma, 409c, 410
Sarcomeres, 13, 17
Sartorius, 8f
    knees, 30c
    synovial joint motions, 27c, 28c
Saturated fats and fatty acids, 197, 209–210, 215
Scales to take weight, 135
Scapula, 32c, 77f, 79, 89
Scar tissue, 401
Schlemm's canal, 347
Schwann cells, 335
Sciatica, 356, 357
    lumbar radiculopathy, 361
    radiculopathy, 360
Science and math abilities, 332f
Sclera, 347

Scoliosis, 100
Seafood, 210
Sebaceous glands, 376f, 380, 391, 392
Seborrhea, 392, 403
Second-degree burns, 395
Seeds, 201, 224
Seeing stars, 57
Seizures (convulsions), 144, 353–354
    heat stroke, 186
    hypoglycemia, 166
Selenium, 218, 219, 227
Semimembranosus, 9f
    legs (hamstrings), 30c
    synovial joint motions, 27c, 28c
Semitendinosus, 9f
    knees, 30c
    legs (hamstrings), 30c
    synovial joint motions, 27c, 28c
Semi vegetarians, 428
Sepsis, 98, 428
Septum, 242f
Serine, 206
Seronegative arthritis, 97
Serratus anterior, 8f
Set-point theory, 152
Sex hormones
    manganese's role with, 226
    sebaceous glands, 380
Sexual arousal, 328
Sexual development, endocrine system's role, 381
Sexual dysfunction, lumbar radiculopathy causing, 361
Shakiness from hypoglycemia, 166
Shellfish
    cholesterol levels, 294

vitamin B-12 from, 294
Shingles (herpes zoster), 393, 400
    confused with thoracic radiculopathy, 361
Shin splints, 61
    compared to stress fractures, 99
Shoes
    caught on irregular surface as cause of ACL tears, 64
    tight fit causing blister, 394
Shortening (saturated fat), 209, 214
Shoulders. See also Rotator cuffs
    abduction, 26c, 33c
    adduction, 26c
    circumduction motion, 90
    coracoacromial arch, 425
    deltoids, 33c. See also Deltoids
    extension, 26c, 32c
    flexion, 33c, 34c
    infraspinatus, 33c
    injuries and conditions
        ankylosing spondylitis, 97
        bursitis, 56
        dislocation, 56
        hyperextension, 56
        shoulder impingement syndrome, 58
    lateral rotation, 26c, 33c
    medial rotation, 26c
    primary joint motions, 33c
    subscapularis, 33c
    supraspinatus, 33c
    synovial joint motions, 25, 26c, 91c
    synovial joints, 85
    teres minor, 33c
    transverse abduction, 26c

transverse adduction, 26c
Shovel use, causing blister, 394
Side vision, 350
Sight. See Vision
Simple carbohydrates, 199, 201
Six-pack. See Body building
Skeletal injuries and conditions, 93–101
    arthritis, 95–98, 96f
    cortisone injections to treat, 101
    kyphosis, 100
    lordosis, 100
    posture abnormalities, 100
    scoliosis, 100
    stress fracture, 99
Skeletal muscles. See Muscular system
Skeletal system, 71–91. See also specific body parts
    anatomical planes, 86, 87f
    appendicular skeleton, 75, 79
    axial skeleton, 75, 78
    bones comprising, 75
    cranium, 78, 80
    diagram with names of bones, 77f
    ears, 81
    face, 81
    frontal (coronal) plane, 86, 87f
        motion on, 88–89
    functions of, 75
    joints. See Joints; Synovial joints
    multiplanar plane motion, 90
    sagittal (lateral) plane, 86, 87f
        motion on, 88, 90
    skull, 80–81
    standard anatomical position, 76
    synovial joint motions. See Synovial joints

transverse (axial) plane, 86, 87f
   motion on, 89–90
vertebral column. *See* Vertebral
   column
Vitamin A's benefits for, 220
Skin
   adipose tissue, 376f, 377
   arrector pili muscle, 376f
   arteries, 376f, 377
   collagen, 378
   conditions, 391–396. *See also* Skin
      conditions and reactions
   connective tissue, 377
   dermis, 376f, 377
   epidermis, 376f, 377
   glands, 377, 379–381. *See also*
      Glands
   hair bulb, 376f
   hair follicles, 376f, 377
   hair shaft, 376f
   hypodermis (subcutaneous), 376f, 377
   keratin, 378
   layers, 376
      diagram of, 376f
   lymph vessels, 377
   melanin, 378
   nerve endings, 376f, 377
   sebaceous glands, 376f, 380, 391, 392
   skin cells, 378
   smooth muscle fibers, 377
   stratum basale, 376f
   stratum corneum, 376f, 394
   stratum granulosum, 376f
   stratum spionsum, 376f

   sweat glands, 376f, 379, 380, 382
   sweat pores, 376f
   veins, 376f, 377
Skin cancer, 392, 409c, 412
Skin cells, 378
Skin color, 378
Skin conditions and reactions, 391–396
   abrasion, 396
   acne, 220, 380, 391
   adhesions, 401
   arthritis as cause of, 97
   athlete's foot (tinea pedis), 392
   avulsion, 396
   bedsores (decubitus ulcer), 394
   blisters (vesicles), 394, 400
   boil (furuncle), 392
   burns, 395
   callus, 394
   carbuncle, 392
   corn (foot), 394
   cosmetic surgery, 404
   dematitis, 391
   dermabrasion, 404
   dry gangrene, 392
   eczema, 392, 400
   erythema, 391
   first-degree burns, 395
   gangrene, 392
   hives (urticaria), 393
   hypertrophic scar tissue, 401
   impetigo, 400
   incision, 396
   keloid scar tissue, 401
   laceration, 396
   large blisters (bullae), 400
   melanoma (skin cancer), 392

nevus (mole or birthmark), 393
postules, 392
psoriasis, 392, 403
puncture, 396
scar tissue, 401
seborrhea, 392, 403
second-degree burns, 395
shingles. *See* Shingles
sunburn, 395
third-degree burns, 395
vitamin B-6 protecting against, 222
vitamin B-7 protecting against, 222
warts, 393
wet gangrene, 392
wounds, 396
Skin layers, 376
diagram of, 376*f*
Skin tags, 125
Skull. *See* Head
Sleep
burning calories during, 147
endocrine system's role, 381
melatonin's role, 380
muscle building and, 203
Sliding filament theory, 13
Slow-twitch red muscle fiber, 10, 11, 23
Slurred speech
concussion, 57
hypoglycemia, 166
stroke symptoms, 296
Small calorie, 191
Small intestine, 108, 108*f*, 109, 110–111, 115
Crohn's disease and, 126
inguinal hernia, 119

umbilical hernia, 120
Smell (sense of)
in aura phase of grand mal seizure, 354
zinc's role, 227
Smell produced by apocrine sweat glands, 382
Smoking
Crohn's disease, risk of, 127
gastroesophageal reflux disease (GERD) and, 129
primary risk factor, 422
stroke, increased risk for, 296
Smooth (visceral) muscles, 6*f*, 7, 377
arteries, 255*f*
veins, 255*f*
Sneezing
autonomic nervous system controlling, 328
function of, 306
medulla controlling, 331
Snellen visual acuity chart, 366
Social recognition and identity, 375, 386
Soda, 201
Sodium, 75, 187, 218, 219, 227
high blood-sodium level (hypernatremia), 187
iodized salt, 226
low blood-sodium level (hyponatremia), 187
Soleus, 8*f*, 9*f*
ankles, 30*c*
synovial joint motions, 28*c*
Soma, 333*f*, 334
Somatotype, 414

Sound (sense of)
    in aura phase of grand mal seizure, 354
    tinnitus, 402
Soybean oil, 212
Soybeans, 212
Spasms
    hypochloremia causing, 186
    lower back pain, 57
    warm-up and cool-down preventing, 181–182, 270
Spastic bowel, 122
Spastic colon, 122
Speech, loss of or difficulties with, 325, 426. *See also* Slurred speech
    stroke symptoms, 296
Speed of movement, 42
Sphenoid bone, 80
Sphenoid sinus, 303f, 304, 305
Sphygmomanometer, 245
Spices, 230
Spinal canal, 327
    vertebral arch around, 340
Spinal cord. *See also* Disks; Vertebrae; Vertebral column
    cauda equina, 341
    in central nervous system, 325, 327, 337
    components of, 337–338
    connection to brain, 327
    injuries and conditions. *See* Nervous system injuries and conditions
    medulla at end of, 331
    membranes, 337
    vitamin B-9 deficiency causing defects in, 223
Spinal stenosis, 340, 356, 358, 359–360
Spine, 337. *See also* Vertebral column
    also called backbone, spinal column, or vertebral column, 337
    injuries and conditions
        ankylosing spondylitis, 97
        kyphosis, 100
        lordosis, 100
        posture abnormalities, 100
        scoliosis, 100
    joints, 85
    Paget's disease, 360
Spondylolisthesis, 357
Spondylosis, 358
Spot reducing exercises, 183
Sprains vs. strains, 55
Squamous cell carcinoma, 409c, 412
Squats
    benefits of, 178
    injuries and conditions common to
        patellofemoral pain syndrome, 63
        torn meniscus (cartilage), 64
Stabilization, 21, 41
Stabilization process, 154–155
Stabilizer muscles, 21
Standard anatomical position, 76
Starches. *See also* Carbohydrates
    digestion of, 114
    food examples, 201
    polysaccharides, 200
Starvation, 143–145
Static stretches, 44–45

active static stretches, 45
passive static stretches, 45, 47
Stationary bicycles, 261
Steps, climbing up
   burning calories, 147
   motor units and, 23
Steriod hormones, 289
Sternocleidonmastoid, 8f
Sternum, 77f, 78
   cartilaginous joints (synchondroses), 85
Stethoscope, 245, 248
Stiffness from arthritis, 95, 97
Still's disease, 97
Stirrup (ear), 81
Stomach, 107, 108, 108f
   fat cells, 138
   gastric juices, 114
   inguinal hernia, 119
   peptic ulcer, 121
   tumors, 121
   visceral muscle in, 7
Stool, 112
Strains vs. sprains, 55
Strangulated hemorrhoid, 125
Stratum basale, 376f
Stratum corneum, 376f
Stratum granulosum, 376f
Stratum spionsum, 376f
Strength training, 13, 17, 151, 269
   best age for strength gain, 17
   circuit training, 269
   large muscle fiber, development of, 24
   maintaining muscle tissue, 150
   motor learning factor, 24

for patellar tendonitis (jumpers knee), 63
for patellofemoral pain syndrome, 63
Stress fractures, confused with shin splints, 61
Stress tests, 261, 263, 271
Stretching, 265, 267
   autogenic inhibition to safeguard against excessive stretching, 51
   compared to contraction and stabilization, 41
   contract/relax method, 47
   defined, 44
   dynamic (ballistic) stretches, 46, 48
   muscular system, 41
   myotatic reflex, 48
   neurophysiological effects of, 48–49
   overstretching (stretch weakness), 65
   proprioceptive neuromuscular facilitation (PNF), 47
   proprioceptors, 49
   safety responses to, 50–51
   static stretch, 44
   types of, 44–47
Stria vascularis, 378
Stroke
   cerebral embolism, 295
   cerebral hemorrhage, 295
   cerebral thrombosis, 295
   cerebrovascular accident (CVA), 295
   emergency care for, 296
   HDL protecting against, 290

range of damage, 296
seizures as result of, 353
symptoms, 296
trans fatty acids increasing risk of, 214
triglycerides increasing risk of, 213
Stroke volume, 250
Stroma, 348
Stunting, 414
Subcutaneous fat, 137
Sublingual glands, 114
Subluxation, 56
Submandibular glands, 114
Subscapularis, 33c
Substrate, 161
Sucrose (table sugar), 199, 201
Suet, 209
Suffocation, 317
Sugar. *See also* Glucose
brown sugar, 201
eating foods with lower sugar, 142
fructose (fruit sugar), 199
galactose (milk sugar), 199
lactose (milk sugar), 199
maltose (malt sugar). *See* Maltose
simple carbohydrates, 199
sucrose (table sugar), 199, 201
white sugar, 201
Suggested daily intakes, 197, 203, 212, 215
Sulfur, 219
Sunburn, 395
Superficial position, 418
Superficial temporal arteries, 248
Superior lobe, 303f, 308
Superior position, 418

Superior rectus muscle, 344f
Superior vena cava, 237f, 239, 242f, 256, 258f
Supination of arm, 34c, 90
Supine, 428
Supplements
coenzyme Q10 (CoQ10) supplements, 229
fish-oil supplements, 212
protein supplements, 204
vitamin D-2, 224
Supra- (position), 418
Supraspinatus, 26c, 33c
Surgeries
arthroscopic surgery, 64
cosmetic surgery, 404
eye conditions, 367–369
Swallowing
medulla controlling, 331
nervous system impairment causing difficulties, 325
stroke symptom of difficulty in swallowing, 296
Sweat glands, 376f, 379, 380, 382
apocrine, 382
eccrine, 382
sudoriferous glands, 382
Sweating
autonomic nervous system controlling, 328
heat exhaustion, 186
hypoglycemia, 166
hyponatremia, 187
Sweat pore, 376f
Swelling, 398
arthritis, 95, 97

edema, 399
hand-foot syndrome, 222
inflammation, 398
RICE techniques for reduction, 66–67
shoulder impingement, 58
synovial fluid, 84
Swimmers
　burning calories, 147
　shoulder impingement syndrome, 58
Swivel (pivot) joint, 91c
Symbols that express quantities of nutrients, 196
　AI (adequate intake), 196
　g (grams), 196
　IU (international units), 196
　mcg (μg) (micrograms), 196
　mg (milligrams), 196
Sympathetic nervous system, 329
Synchondroses (cartilaginous joints), 85
Syncope. See Fainting or feeling faint
Syndesmoses (fibrous joints), 85
Synergist muscle, 22
Synovial fluid, 84
Synovial joints (diarthroses), 26–28c, 85
　ball & socket joint, 91c
　ellipsiod (condyloid) joint, 91c
　gliding (planar) joint, 91c
　hinge joint, 91c
　mechanics of, 91c
　meniscus, 37
　motions, 25, 26–28c, 88–90, 91c
　　abduction, 89
　　adduction, 88
　　circumduction, 90

depression, 89
dorsiflexion, 90
elevation, 89
eversion, 90
extension, 88
flexion, 88
horizontal extension, 89
horizontal flexion, 89
inversion, 90
opposition, 90
plantar flexion, 90
pronation, 90
rotary motion, 89
rotation, 89
supination, 90
　normal joint vs. osteoarthritis, 96f
　pivot (swivel) joint, 91c
　saddle joint, 91c
　synovial fluid, 84
Synovial membrane, 358
Synovitis, 358
Synovium, 340, 358
Synthesis, 162, 428
Syrup, 201
Systemic disease, 428
System integration, 131–230
　body building, 175–188. See also Body building
　body composition, 133–173. See also Body composition
Systolic blood pressure, 246, 247

T

Table sugar (sucrose), 199, 201
Talk test, 272
Tallow, 209

Tarsals, 77f, 79, 91c
Taste (sense of)
    in aura phase of grand mal seizure, 354
    zinc's role, 227
Tea, 230
Teamwork approach to stretching, 47
Tearing
    of meniscus, 37, 64
    of muscle or connective tissue, 46
Tears, 346
Teeth, 114
    calcium's role, 225
    fluoride's role, 226
    number of, 114
    phosphorus's role, 227
    protection from saliva, 113
TEF (thermal effect of food), 153
Temporal bones, 80
Temporal pulse site, 248
Tendon, 7, 14f, 36
    Achilles tendon, 62
    aponeurosis, 36
    epimysium tendons, 14f, 15
    injuries and conditions. *See also* Tendonitis
        biceps tendon rupture, 58
        rupture, 56, 62, 63
        strains, 55
    insertion, location of, 21
Tendon insertion, 21
Tendonitis, 56
    Achilles tendonitis, 62
    patellar tendonitis (jumpers knee), 63
Tennis elbow (epicondylitis), 58

Tennis players
    shoulder impingement syndrome, 58
    tennis elbow (epicondylitis), 58
Tensor fasciae latae, 8f, 27c
Teres major, 9f, 26c
Teres minor, 26c, 33c
Tests. *See* Diagnostic tests and tools
Therapeutic angiogenesis, 428
Thermal effect of food (TEF), 153
Thiamine (vitamin B-1), 217, 221
Thinking, 331, 332f
Third-degree burns, 395
Thorac- (body part designation), 417
Thoracic cavity, 239
Thoracic radiculopathy, 361
Thoracic vertebrae, 82f, 83, 419
Thoraco-lumbar fascia, 9f
Threonine, 206
Throat. *See* Pharynx
Thrombocytes, 428. *See* Platelets
THRR (training heart rate range), 273
Thumb motion, 90, 91c
Thyroid
    iodine's role, 226
    location, 157
    overactive (hyperthyroidism), 157
    selenium's role, 227
    underactive (hypothyroidism), 157
Tibia, 77f, 79
    shin splints, 61
Tibialis. *See* Anterior tibialis; Posterior tibialis
Tingling
    cervical radiculopathy causing, 361
    radiculopathy causing, 357, 360

seizures causing, 353
Tissue cell abnormalities, 407–416
    cancer. *See* Cancer
Toe nails, 387
Tongue, salivary glands under, 114
Tonometry, 365
Torn mensicus or cartilage, 37, 64
Total blood cholesterol, 291, 292*c*
Total fat intake, 215
Trabecular meshwork, 347
Trace minerals, 219
Trachea (windpipe), 303*f*, 304, 305, 307–309
Training heart rate range (THRR), 273
Trans fatty acids, 210, 214
Transverse abdominis, 31*c*
    workout chart, 180*c*
Transverse abduction, 26*c*
Transverse adduction, 26*c*
Transverse (axial) plane, 86, 87*f*
    motion on, 89–90
Trapezius muscles, 8*f*, 9*f*, 32*c*, 89
Trauma, 359
Treadmills, 261
Tretinoin, 220
Tri- (anatomical number three), 420
Triceps, 9*f*, 21
    primary joint motions, 34*c*
    skeletal muscles, 26*c*
    synovial joint motions, 26*c*
    workout chart, 180*c*
Triceps brachii, 34*c*
Triglycerides, 208, 212, 213, 291. *See also* Lipoproteins
    range references, 292*c*
Tryptophan, 206

Tumor (neoplasm), 409*c*, 411
Tumors of the spine, 359
Tunnel vision, 363
Twitching, seizures causing, 353
Type 1 diabetes, 165
Type 1 muscle fiber, 11
Type 2 diabetes, 166
    BMI as factor, 169
Type 2 muscle fiber, 10
Tyrosine, 206

U

Ulcerative colitis, 126
Ulcers
    bulimia causing, 146
    Crohn's disease and, 127
    peptic ulcer, 121
Ulna, 77*f*, 79
    fibrous joints (syndesmoses), 85
Umbilical hernia, 120
Unconsciousness, 57, 328, 331, 354, 375
Undercorrection, 369
Underweight, in body mass index (BMI), 172*c*
Unmyelinated and myelinated axons, 335
Unsaturation, 210
Unsubtyped IBS (IBS-U), 122
Upper GI tract, 107–108
Upper heart chambers, 241
Upper respiratory tract, 304, 305–306
Upper trapezius, 32*c*
Uric acid, 98
Urinary tract infections, 146
Urination, autonomic nervous system controlling, 328

Urticaria (hives), 393
Uvea (uveal tract), 345, 347

V
Valine, 206
Valsalva maneuver, 319, 428
Valve, 255f
Vasovagal reaction, 428
Vastus intermedius
    legs (quadriceps), 22, 30c
    synovial joint motions, 28c
Vastus lateralis, 8f, 9f
    legs (quadriceps), 22, 30c
    synovial joint motions, 28c
Vastus medialis, 8f
    legs (quadriceps), 22, 30c
    synovial joint motions, 28c
Vegans, 428
Vegetable oils, 209, 224
Vegetables. *See* Fruits and vegetables
Vegetable shortening, 214
Vegetarians, 428
    lacto, 428
    lacto-ovo, 428
    ovo, 428
    pesco, 428
    semi, 428
Veins, 236, 237f, 257
    compared to arteries, 255
    diagram of, 255f
    femoral vein, 258f
    function of, 257
    great saphenous vein, 258f
    iliac vein, 258f
    inner layer, 255f
    jugular vein, 258f
    outer layer, 255f
    posterior tibial vein, 258f
    pulmonary veins, 237f, 239, 242f, 257, 258f, 310
    renal vein, 258f
    skin and, 376f, 377
    smooth muscle, 255f
    valve, 255f
    venous system, 256
    venules, 257
Vena cava, 237f, 239, 242f, 256, 258f
Venous system, 255, 256
Ventral position, 418
Ventricles
    brain, 330f
    heart, 237f, 241, 242f, 250
Venules, 257
Vertebrae, 327, 337
    cervical vertebrae, 82f, 83, 419
    coccyx, 82f, 83
    facet joints, 340
    intervertebral foramen (neural foramen), 340
    lamina, 340
    ligaments, 340
    ligamentum flavum, 340
    lumbar vertebrae, 82f, 83, 419
    pedicles, 340
    sacrum, 82f, 83
    synovium, 340
    thoracic vertebrae, 82f, 83, 419
Vertebral arch, 340
Vertebral column, 78, 82f, 83, 338. *See also* Spine; Vertebrae
    cervical vertebrae, 82f, 83, 419
    coccyx, 82f, 83

diagram of, 82f
function of, 83
lumbar vertebrae, 82f, 83, 419
sacrum, 82f, 83
thoracic vertebrae, 82f, 83, 419
Vesicles (blisters), 394, 400
Violent sports. *See also* Boxers; Football players
concussion risk, 57
Virus
blisters associated with diseases, 400
warts, 393
Visceral fat, 137
Visceral muscles, 7
Visceral nervous system. *See* Autoniomic nervous system
Viscous property (or plastic elongation deformation), 43
Vision, 331, 342
accommodation, 349, 363
acuity, 350, 363
binocular vision, 349
central vision, 350
color vision, 346
contrast sensitivity, 349
diabetes causing blindness, 165
farsightedness, 363
legal blindness, 363
low vision, 363
nearsightedness, 363
peripheral vision, 350
side vision, 350
tunnel vision, 363
visual field, 350
Vitamin A's benefits for, 220

vitamin B-7 protective powers, 222
Visual acuity, 350, 363
Visual disturbance as symptom of stroke, 296
Visual field, 350
Vitamin A (retinol), 217, 218, 220, 228
Vitamin A acid (also called all-trans-retinoic acid, ATRA, retinoic acid, or Tretinoin), 220
Vitamin B-1 (thiamine), 217, 218, 221
Vitamin B-2 (riboflavin), 217, 218, 221
Vitamin B-3 (niacin), 217, 218, 221
Vitamin B-5 (pantothenic acid), 217, 218, 222
Vitamin B-6 (pyridoxine), 217, 218, 222
Vitamin B-7 (biotin), 217, 218, 222
Vitamin B-9 (folic acid), 217, 218, 223
Vitamin B-12 (cobalamin), 217, 218, 223
Vitamin C (ascorbic acid), 217, 218, 223, 228
Vitamin D (cholecalciferol), 217, 218, 224
Vitamin D-2, 224
Vitamin D-3, 224
Vitamin E (alpha-tocopherol), 217, 218, 224, 228
Vitamin H. *See* Vitamin B-7
Vitamin K, 217, 218, 224
Vitamin K1 (phytonadione), 224
Vitamin K2, 224
Vitamins, 193, 195, 217–224. *See also specific types*
descriptions, 220–224
essential vitamins, 217
fat-soluble, 207, 218, 220
list of types of, 217

water-soluble, 195, 221–223
Vitreous gel, 344f
Vitreous humor, 344, 347
VO2 Max, 263
Voice. *See also* Speech, loss of or difficulties with
dysphonia, 426
Voice box (larynx), 303f, 304, 305
Volleyball players, injuries and conditions common to
Achilles tendonitis and rupture, 62
patellar tendonitis (jumpers knee), 63
Voluntary actions, 325
Voluntary muscles. *See* Muscular system
Vomer bones, 81
Vomiting (emesis)
autonomic nervous system controlling, 328
bulimia, 146
concussion, 57
definition of, 426
heat exhaustion, 186
hypochloremia resulting from, 186
hypokalemia caused by, 156

W

Waist size. *See* Body building
Warm-ups and cool-downs, 181–182, 265, 266, 270
Warnings. *See also* Physicians, consultation of
ballistic stretching, 46
blisters, not to burst, 400
holding your breath while exercising, 319

protein consumption, when excessive, 197, 204
stroke, need for immediate medical care, 296
training at or near 90 percent of maximum heart rate, 281
vitamin dosage, when excessive, 218, 221
Warts, 393
Waste removal
from cells, 235, 238, 290–291
from digestion, 112, 115
plasma's role in, 252
respiratory system's role in, 301, 305
Water consumption
benefits of, 198
daily amount, 139, 198
exercise requirements, 198
fasting and, 144
flavored water, 201
functions of, 198
hyponatremia, 187
muscle tissue, water and protein composition of, 203
water as nutrient, 195
Water-soluble vitamins, 195, 221–223
Wavefront, 366
Weather conditions, 185
Weight. *See* Body composition; Weight gain; Weight loss
Weight gain. *See also* Calories
basal metabolic rate (BMR) as factor in, 159
Weight lifting. *See also* Body building
abdominal definition (building six-pack), 184

benefit of increasing basal metabolic rate (BMR), 160
compared to aerobic exercise
adding muscle, 158
calorie burning, 147–148
fast-twitch muscle fiber, 10
in fitness program, 140
injuries and conditions common to
shoulder impingement syndrome, 58
tennis elbow (epicondylitis), 58
torn meniscus (cartilage), 64
protein supplements, 204
Weight loss. See also Calories
exercise
calorie burning comparison, 147–148
importance of, 140, 142
training heart rate range (THRR), 273
extreme weight loss resulting in anorexia nervosa, 143
fasting, 144
fat loss and, 135, 139
to lose one to two pounds per week, 141
recommended methods, 142
reducing daily caloric intake, 139, 141
spot reducing exercises, 183
Weight of brain, 331
Weight training. See Body building
Wet gangrene, 392
Wheat, 201
Wheezing, 318
White blood cells (leukocytes), 75, 251, 253
abnormal number resulting in leukemia. See Leukemia
White coat hypertension, 247
White fat cells, 138
White sugar, 201
Whole grains. See Grains
Windpipe. See Trachea
Wolff's Law, 188
Women. See Male vs. female; Mammary glands; Menstrual cycle; Pregnancy
Workouts. See Aerobic exercises; Body building; *specific types of exercises*
Wounds, 396
Wrists
extensor carpi radialis, 9f, 35c
extensor carpi ulnaris, 9f, 35c
flexor carpi radialis, 8f, 9f, 35c
flexor carpi ulnaris, 35c
primary joint motions, 35c
radial pulse site, 248
rheumatoid arthritis, 97
skeletal muscles, 35c
synovial joints, 91c
Writing ability, 332f

Y

Yeast, 221–224
Yogurt, 201
Yo-yo effect (weight loss), 146

Z

Zinc, 218, 219, 227
Zollinger-Ellison syndrome, 121
Zonules, 348
Zygomatic bones, 81

Warning

- Always consult a doctor before beginning any exercise program.

- We urge you to have a certified professional fitness trainer to assist you with your exercise program.

- Common sense must always prevail when selecting exercises and their frequency, duration, and intensity.

- When you exercise, common sense must always prevail when addressing extrinsic factors such as weather conditions, clothing, footwear, terrain, water supply, food eaten or available, workout partners, or any other conditions outside of your body that have the potential to affect your body adversely.

- The contents of this book are not intended to provide personal exercises, eating programs, or medical advice to you, or any person or persons, whatsoever.

- This book is intended to provide scholastic information for educational use, and to provide the awareness that there may be a need for medical supervision and/or guidance by a certified professional fitness trainer whenever a fitness program of any kind is desired. With this warning, the author assumes no responsibility whatsoever for a medical event of any kind, injury, or damages to persons or property.

- The use of any or all information herein should first be approved by the appropriate medical professional.

Speed Learning for Anatomy
Systems and Functions of the Human Body
Quick and Easy
Vol. 02-JCB
Copyright ©

Author: Justina C. Bachsteiner PhD

Editor: Justina C. Bachsteiner PhD

Editor: Adam W. Rossly Sr.

All copyright laws for intellectual property apply.

This edited version is from the 2002 Copyrighted © "Super Health Tips Glossary."